BREATHING
EASY

BREATHING
EASY

✿ ✿ ✿

A Parent's Guide to Dealing with Your Child's Asthma

Maryann Stevens

PRENTICE
HALL
PRESS

New York   London   Toronto   Sydney   Tokyo   Singapore

For Pamela, David, and Melissa

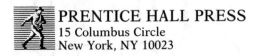

PRENTICE HALL PRESS
15 Columbus Circle
New York, NY 10023

PRENTICE HALL PRESS and colophons are registered
trademarks of Simon & Schuster, Inc.

Library of Congress Cataloging-in-Publication Data

Stevens, Maryann.
  Breathing easy : a parent's guide to dealing with your
child's asthma/Maryann Stevens.
  Includes index.
  ISBN 0–13–083692-3
  1. Asthma in children—popular works. I. Title.
RJ436.A8574 1991
618.92'238-dc20   90-25564
                                                        CIP

Manufactured in the United States of America

10 9 8 7 6 5 4 3 2 1

First Edition

The following organizations have generously given their permission to use information provided by them: American Lung
Association (National Office), 1740 Broadway, New York, NY,
10019–4374; Asthma & Allergy Foundation of America; the National Asthma Education Program of the Department of Health &
Human Services; Johns Hopkins Children's Center; Mothers of
Asthmatics, Inc.

ACKNOWLEDGMENTS

This book could not have been written without the advice and wisdom of Dr. R. Michael Sly of Children's National Medical Center in Washington, DC. Our "St. Michael" has dedicated his career to our wheezing children. I can never thank him enough. He really cares about every wheeze, hive, and unknown rash. Dr. Sly never hurries the parent and is willing to answer countless questions. He listens to the teenager who sometimes only relates his dread between the lines of a glib remark. He never rebukes or passes judgment on parent or child, and he makes our asthmatics *well*. If I were asked to describe the perfect doctor it would be Dr. R. Michael Sly.

I would also like to thank Judy Hines, whose question "Would you like to write a book?" inspired my literary efforts. Without her editing and good humor, this project would never have seen completion. She was my roommate at Duke and has been my best friend throughout the years. Her own family experiences with asthma added greatly to this book.

Heartfelt thanks, too, to Dr. Lawrence J. Murphy of Burke, Virginia, for his guidance and instruction, and for the confidence he had in me during my "learning years" in his office. Of course, no list would be complete without a special thank you to my very first mentor, Dr. Frank J. Murphy, now of Hilton Head, South Carolina—a very special person who not only cared for the physical ills of his patients but understood the spiritual needs and values so necessary to healing.

I want also to thank Mary Lou Sheehan and Helen Middleton, allergy nurses who shared their knowledge and experiences with me. Among the many mothers who have shared their experiences, I would like to thank Terri Dickerson-Jones and Dorothy Baumgartner.

This book is a result of many people who had faith in the project. Debbie Romash, Richard Cramer, Flip Brophy, and Gail Winston really offered the support and practical advice that made it happen.

My children and I have been blessed with a father and husband who believed from the first wheeze that everything would be all right. Whatever fears he might have had, he never transmitted them to us. We have turned to him for guidance, reassurance, and emotional support time and time again. He has never let us down. Gary is our secret weapon, our Rock of Gibraltar, our port in all storms. We love him very much, and I take full credit for having married him.

CONTENTS

PREFACE

Of the several books on asthma written for the general public, none has been written with the wit and understanding that Maryann Stevens brings to the subject. As the mother of three children who have had severe asthma, she offers practical approaches to the problems of raising a youngster with asthma. You will find her suggestions not only helpful but possibly lifesaving.

More than thirty-five hundred people have died from asthma each year in the United States since 1983. This figure includes more than a hundred children each year. As recently as 1977, only fifty-four children died from the disease. Although the death rate from asthma remains low in comparison to such an illness as heart disease, the doubling of the rate within six years and its continued increase are of major concern.

We estimate that between 3 percent and 5 percent of people in the United States probably have asthma, and 10 percent to 15 percent of children have had it at some time. While numbers of deaths make news, they actually underestimate the importance of asthma as a cause of illness. Asthma accounts for nearly one fourth of the time lost from school due to chronic illness.

The greatest tragedy of the recent increases in deaths from asthma is that most of these fatalities probably could have been prevented. What can you do for your children to protect them from the worst consequences of asthma?

1. First, find out whether your child really has asthma. It may be just as important to discover he doesn't, because some other condition that may require immediate treatment could be causing his wheezing. Among them could be the aspiration of a peanut or another object by a toddler. If your physician is unable to find the cause of recurrent coughing, wheezing, and difficult breathing, ask for referral to an allergist or lung disease specialist.

2. Find out what causes asthma in your child. You probably know that strenuous exercise, cigarette smoke, and respiratory infections are causes. If symptoms get worse in the autumn, your child may be allergic to ragweed pollen. An allergist can determine through skin testing whether your child has an allergy to pollens, molds, animals, or house dust.

3. Avoid causes of asthma or try to minimize their effects. Do not permit smoking in your home and ask to be seated in the no smoking areas at restaurants.

Simple precautions such as eliminating carpet from the bedroom greatly reduce exposure to house dust.

If your child has a bad reaction to aspirin, avoid related drugs like ibuprofen and indomethacin. In fact, avoid any drug that contains aspirin. If your child has a sensitivity to sulfites, avoid any food that may contain them.

Have your child inhale a beta agonist such as albuterol (see chapter 4 for more details on this drug and others named in this Preface) before he does any strenuous exercise. By inhaling cromolyn, he can protect himself against the unavoidable, brief exposure to allergens such as pollen or cat fur.

Allergy injections are helpful for children who are allergic to pollens and molds, but don't expect improvement until months of treatment have passed.

4. Follow your physician's recommendations for medications. If you don't understand them, ask for a more complete explanation and request them in writing. Know when your child should take the medicine, how he should take it, and what are the possible side effects. Know how to contact your physician if the medicine is not effective or if side effects occur. Know whom to contact when your regular physician is not available.

5. Understand exactly how to use any inhaler prescribed for your youngster. Ask the physician or nurse to demonstrate its use and to watch your child use it. Written instructions cannot substitute adequately for demonstration. Know how long to expect improvement to continue after treatment with a beta-agonist. Contact your physician whenever increasingly frequent use of the inhaler is needed. If moderate to

xiv

moderately severe wheezing fails to improve after inhalation of the beta-agonist, the child has not used the inhaler properly or the drug is no longer effective and different treatment is needed. Contact the physician or go to an emergency room immediately.

6. Ask your physician whether you or your child should be instructed in giving an injection of epinephrine or terbutaline. It may be necessary in the event of any emergency when severe asthma may prevent adequate inhalation of a beta-agonist.

7. Don't disregard symptoms. Use the prescribed medication immediately. Response is best to medication taken when symptoms begin.

8. Learn all you can about asthma from this book and the reliable sources mentioned in it—among them the Asthma and Allergy Foundation of America, 1717 Massachusetts Ave., N.W., Suite 305, Washington, DC 20036; the American Lung Association, 1740 Broadway, New York, NY 10019; and Mothers of Asthmatics, Inc., 10875 Main St., Suite 210, Fairfax, VA 22030.

—*R. Michael Sly, M.D.*
Director, Allergy and Immunology
Department, Children's National
Medical Center, and Professor of
Pediatrics, The George Washington
University School of Medicine and
Health Sciences

INTRODUCTION

"Eventually, everyone becomes an expert on some subject," said a close friend of mine when we were both young mothers. We were suffering from stay-at-home, no-growth blues, and I adopted this philosophy instantly, eager to dream of a more illustrious future. What would it be? Politics? A sport? Writing a great novel?

Little did I suspect that my future field of expertise would announce itself with a wheeze. The wheeze came from my fourteen-month-old daughter, Pamela, who was followed in sequence by her brother, David, and sister, Melissa. All three children developed severe asthma.

In the beginning I knew nothing about the disease, and had no idea how to handle it. I lived in anguish, waiting for the next emergency, terrified that each episode of torturous breathing would end in catastrophe. It was no way to live.

I realized that if our family was going to control the children's asthma, I had to understand all aspects of the disease: the known causes, the changes it produces in the body, and the recommended medications and their purposes. Once I learned about the enemy, I could start controlling it. As time passed, I became more confident in my ability to handle this chronic illness.

Nine years ago I took an administrative position with my children's local pediatricians. I had no formal medical training, having majored in political science at Duke University, but I thought it would be a good opportunity to learn more about general healthcare. Over the eight years I was associated with these fine doctors, I mastered and performed almost all of the nursing skills and techniques required by the practice (all of these procedures were done under the doctors' supervision).

More important, in dealing with the many asthmatic children served by the practice, I observed the same anxieties on the part of other parents that I had experienced and conquered. Dr. Frank J. Murphy, who started this practice and is now retired, encouraged me to develop and teach a class for asthmatic children and their parents. I led this class for five years, working with more than two hundred members of families dealing with childhood asthma. I found the moral and informative support I could give was just what the doctor ordered.

The purpose of this book is to provide the same kind of support to other families. The chapters of

Breathing Easy are organized to answer primary questions about the disease first, then provide suggestions for control of asthma on a daily basis—at home, in school, traveling, and in emergencies.

My experience, both clinically and as a parent, has taught me a great deal. I want to share what I have learned with you.

The Stevens Family . . . Asthma and All

Fear is an emotion you can control. You can refuse to recognize it, push it away, conquer it, ignore it. Terror is different. It is alive. It takes over within moments. It invades your body like an electric shock.

I know what terror is. In June 1984, my husband, Gary, and I experienced it as we watched our thirteen-year-old daughter, air-hungry, strangling, her eyes rolling and unfocused, an awful gurgling sound rising in her throat. We could witness it, but we couldn't intervene. The specialized personnel of the intensive care unit, white-coated strangers, surrounded her. She needed us so very much, but we couldn't help her.

We had never seen a respirator before, but when one was wheeled in front of us in the intensive care unit, we knew instantly what it was. The medical staff closed the door, left us outside, and the terror isolated us from Melissa and from each other.

Asthma was an old enemy. We had fought it for more than twenty years. We had learned to understand it and, in two of our children, control it. Now, with the youngest experiencing acute episodes that were intensifying with each passing year, the battle was escalating, but we were far from giving up

FACING THE CHALLENGE

Meet Pamela (age twenty-five), David (age twenty-two), and Melissa (age fifteen) Stevens. Together they can account for a combined total of forty-five years of our family's fight against asthma. We have made more than forty hospital visits, and spent at least five thousand hours in doctors' offices. We have purchased enough medication and machinery to outfit a clinic.

But those statistics don't represent who these three young people are. They are, in fact, three wonderful individuals who have overcome a chronic disease that has ranged from bothersome to life-threatening. Today they are leading full, exciting lives, enriched because they have learned so much from challenging and beating asthma.

When Pamela and David were little, we didn't know what to expect, and there was no place to look to get the answers we wanted to the basic questions about asthma. We had to learn the hard way—a little bit here, a little bit there.

By the time Melissa came along (ten years after Pamela), at least we understood the dynamics of the disease, although her case was different from her brother and sister's. We knew the causes and treatments and the reasons for them, and as parents, this knowledge helped us cope successfully with the ups and downs that a child with asthma experiences.

Keeping Calm

Pamela had her first asthma attack when she was just over a year old. When we arrived at the hospital facing the possibility of her having a tracheotomy, Gary and I were visibly upset. Our daughter's pediatrician told us that if she had broken her leg our emotional upset wouldn't make any real difference to her. But she didn't have a simple broken leg; she had a chronic disease.

Although asthma is not caused by emotions, it can be affected by them. An asthma attack may be intensified if the child becomes upset. Pamela's doctor warned us that our child would look to us to find out whether she was all right or not. As we reacted, she would read our faces to know whether she should be frightened. We couldn't afford the luxury of being emotional.

This advice was about the best we ever received. From that time on, both Gary and I realized it was up to us to set the tone. If the children knew we weren't upset, that we could take a mild or even an acute attack in stride, then they could too.

FAMILY STRENGTHS

You'll also want to know the parents in the Stevens family. Not because we're extraordinary people. We're not. But from that first time we faced what was ahead of us with asthma, we have built on our individual strengths to face the disease. When one of us fell down, the other was ready to fill the gap.

Gary is, by nature, ready to face even the worst situation with solid equanimity. I am more excitable, more volatile. He has helped me learn to curb my emotions when emergency situations (or long-term frustrations) have tested my elasticity.

I have been willing and able to pay attention to the most minute details of therapeutic treatment for asthma in all three children, to the point of literally making a career out of learning about the disease and its treatment. I'm inclined to become totally absorbed in any subject that interests me, and certainly asthma has become my obsession. Gary is less of a detail man. He appreciates the time and attention I give to all aspects of asthma, and defers to me as the expert.

I am the talkative one, the family philosopher. I'm willing to confront anyone and everyone, if necessary, to get what my children need in the way of information, diagnosis, and treatment. I preach without embarrassment about the ideals and attitudes I believe must operate within individuals and families facing adversity. On the other hand, I'll do almost anything for a laugh, to keep the family's good humor in working order. Gary, in his quiet way, sees to it that the family organization operates as smoothly and efficiently as possible.

Enough about our personalities. It is all just to say that whatever traits are mixed and matched among parents and children, they can be blended together to fight asthma. So rely on your strengths, as a single parent or a couple, in dealing with your child's disease, and you'll operate more effectively.

DRAMATIC ENCOUNTERS

I remember when Pamela was about seven or eight years old, and was going to be in the school play. I no longer remember what it was about, but I do remember that the players' burlap costumes were to be supplied by the school, and the parents of the children in the skit were responsible for finding "authentic Israelite sandals."

The play was the most important function of that school year, involving many, many rehearsals. And it became a cause célèbre to find authentic Israelite sandals, especially in the middle of winter, and especially since no one knew what authentic Israelite sandals actually looked like. We had many intense weeks of shopping before we found a pair we thought was authentic enough.

Gary was out of town on the day of the play, so I was responsible for taking Pamela and her very reluctant younger brother to the school auditorium. We parked in the middle of a field next to the school. Pamela ran to join the other thespians enthusiastically. Sure enough, she made a spectacular appearance in her burlap clothing and authentic Israelite sandals.

It wasn't long after her performance, though, that I was called backstage by a frightened teacher. Pamela had broken out in horrendous hives and was wheezing badly. It turned out that she was allergic to the burlap.

David, who had entered the theater so unwillingly, was equally displeased at being forced to leave. I walked out with a wailing little boy in one hand and a mass of wheezing red welts lifted on my other arm, trying to find the car in the dark in the middle of a muddy parking field. Off to the hospital we went for a shot of adrenaline.

To this day, Pamela remembers the play and the thrill of being in it. As an afterthought, she remembers being allergic to the burlap.

This is the way we've tried to bring up our children. They only have one childhood, and Gary and I decided it was going to be as normal for them as possible. Very few times have we not done something, or not let them participate in an activity, because of their asthma. Whatever limitations asthma has put on participation have been defined by letting them try first. We don't anticipate problems before they occur.

Outdoor Types

David, who has always loved the outdoors, spent many weekends with his father—rock climbing, fishing, hiking—even as a little boy. He went out in snow storms; he jumped in every puddle. We had a stream near one of our early homes, and he had a small plastic boat with paddles. He and his friends would paddle up and down that stream for hours.

When David looks back on growing up, he remembers all those wonderful outdoor times. The fact that a lot of them were followed by wheezing is beside the point to him. He remembers the action and the fun.

When Melissa became a Girl Scout, she happened to join a troop whose members were interested in camping. Now, my idea of camping is a motel without a raw bar. But because Melissa wanted to go camping so much, I went with her on one occasion, and Gary went with her on another. Those camping trips featured sleeping outdoors in sleeping bags and/or tents, and tromping through unknown flora and fauna. As this kind of activity could easily trigger an asthma attack, we felt one of us should be there in case we had to get medical help fast.

I can't claim that I became an intrepid camper, but it was a delightful weekend, one that Melissa and I enjoyed thoroughly. And Gary loved his father/daughter weekend, too. To this day, both of us treasure the experiences we had on those trips. And the leaders enjoyed having extra parental participation. Our presence made Melissa just another camper, not one who caused special concern or represented some frightening responsibility they weren't prepared to handle.

Just Another Day in the Life of an Asthmatic

When Melissa started seventh grade, she was attending a brand new school. She had been in school only one week, and I had not had a chance to set up our usual school procedures (see chapter 9). She had a sudden mucus plug and bronchospasm, and couldn't breathe. The school immediately called the rescue squad, and then got in touch with me. They told me the rescue squad was there, but they weren't going to transport her, and that she was feeling much better. I told them I would get there right away. I worked close to Melissa's school, and when I arrived and met the person waiting for me, we walked over to the building she was in. One of her friends, who was watching from the window, turned to the group and said, "Here comes Melissa's mother, and she's smiling." Well, I wasn't smiling because of a nonchalant attitude. My heart was breaking to think that my daughter had to have this happen the very first week of a new school year. But I knew that if the teachers, the principal, and the other children saw that I was handling this situation calmly, they would relax and think this problem wasn't such a big deal after all.

Don't Fence Them In

Over the years, all three of our children have said, at one time or another, "Boy, you're not like other parents. I'm really lucky that you look at things the way you do." I think that's because we learned our priorities very early. We haven't concentrated on the small things that so often impede the relationship between parent and child. Our children know that we won't try to take over their lives. When there have been decisions to be made, it is their feelings we have taken into consideration. We feel that life is about making decisions. In order for children to have enough experience to make really good decisions as they grow older, they need to start making choices when they are young.

Sometimes the decisions our children made didn't work out; they would have an asthma attack in the middle of something they were attempting to do. But they always knew that was all right. We were there with them and would get medical help if needed. They would soon be back on the road again.

The worst thing you can do to a child with asthma is to become overprotective. The damage done in this case is usually not out of unkindness but out of love. If you value your relationship with your child, whether he has asthma or not, it is important to know when to step back. It is a delicate balancing act, because as the parent of an asthmatic you must provide a support system. You must be physically available (a phone call away with transportation to get you to your child immediately), and you must be able to provide the emotional and practical support to let other people who are going to be involved with your child—teachers, scout leaders, coaches, substitute caregivers—know that you can be reached at any time, that the responsibility for your child's illness is never going to fall on them.

You do not have to actually be on the scene at all times. Just the opposite: Your child must feel independent and be able to take part in activities separate from you. However, these activities are most successful when both your child and the adult leaders know you can be reached right away if problems develop. By giving this kind of support, you free other adults from viewing your child as different or frightening. And your child doesn't see himself that way, either.

> *I like to think that my friends feel more comfortable with illness, hospitals, and medication after knowing me. I try to have a sense of humor about asthma. I have also developed a very positive outlook. I try to make the best out of bad situations. I've learned to be more responsible and dependable, especially to myself. I have to be, because I know that I could die from asthma if I do not take a vested interest in regulating it.*
>
> *—MELISSA*

HAPPY ENDINGS

At a good-bye party in our house, one of the neighborhood fathers once said, "I will always remember Pamela running down the street with her petticoats flying, and you flying right behind her." It was about that time one of our doctors told us Pamela would probably never reach adulthood, and if she did she would be emphysemic and probably never lead a normal life. We never believed it, and we never lived that way. We sought new treatments and found a specialist with a different viewpoint. Now Pamela is a trip coordinator for presidential advance at the White House, and is literally flying all over the world.

David was allergic to everything that grew outside. If he did anything outdoors, especially if the weather was uncertain, he was guaranteed to have problems with asthma. He is now a horticulture major. The trees and fruits and flowers—all the things that caused him such difficulty as a child—are his vocation. He has hiked and camped all over the country, and he has no problems with his asthma.

In spring 1984, Melissa was admitted to the intensive care unit of our local hospital twice with asthma attacks that did not seem serious, but ones we had failed to break at home. Both times the attacks took on extremely serious dimensions soon after she arrived at the hospital, the second time resulting in that terrifying introduction to a respirator.

Although she was being treated by a fine team of physicians, several with a special interest in allergies, we agreed with them that the time had come to find a specialist who wrote the medical books on asthma. That person turned out to be Dr. R. Michael Sly at Children's Hospital in Washington, D.C. (known now to all my family and friends as "St. Michael").

Within a month of Dr. Sly's initial workup with

Melissa, and changes in medication based on that workup, Melissa was totally turned around. She was off steroids, which are so often needed in cases of severe chronic asthma, for the first time in several years. She has had only one episode of serious wheezing in more than eighteen months and attends college thanks to Dr. Sly's care.

For the first time since our honeymoon twenty-six years ago, Gary and I were able to take a two-week trip away from the children this year. We felt so sure that Melissa's problems were behind her that we went to Alaska—by boat! Melissa went to visit my sister. She went shopping in New York City amidst all the pollution. And even when she went to her aunt's summer house on the end of Long Island, with ocean breezes and early-morning dews, she had no problems at all.

And what about my own life? Its path takes me back to one of my favorite games when I was a little girl—"follow the dots." After drawing meandering lines along a circuitous route, suddenly a hippopotamus, or a cherry tree, or perhaps Abraham Lincoln, emerged. Life is much the same. Nothing proceeds as the crow flies.

My major in college was political science. My ultimate desire was to be on staff at the White House. For many years that dream was on indefinite hold, as the demands of raising three chronically ill children took precedence. However, over the years I never lost my interest in politics. I volunteered my services for stuffing envelopes, making phone calls, whatever was necessary. I also read extensively. Reading not only brought me knowledge of the world around me but also helped me keep my own problems in perspective. I was able to escape into another landscape when my own was bleak.

My circuitous route took me completely out of politics and into a doctor's office. I learned a great deal about an area that was new to me, and my experience helped me write this book. However, once my children's wheezes were totally under control I saw my dream come true. I volunteered at the White House and eventually came on staff.

We have had three children with severe asthma. Two have no problems anymore, and the third is on her way to good control. Most important, none of them has any emotional scars because of his or her condition. Other children and families can meet the challenge of asthma with the same success. The right attitude plus some knowledge of effective techniques is all it takes.

2

✿ ✿ ✿

Asthma:
Questions and Answers

When our first child's asthma was diagnosed, I knew absolutely nothing about the disease. I thought it had something to do with sneezing. Although my husband, Gary, had experienced asthmatic episodes as a child, and had many relatives with asthma, he had no clear definition of what asthma was or what caused it either. The medical literature we consulted was far too technical for us to understand. There was, in fact, no one reference we could turn to for answers to our questions. Perhaps this chapter will save you a little of the searching and sense of ignorance we suffered.

What is asthma?

The exact abnormality that causes asthma is unknown, but it is known that certain things can act as *triggers*, producing chemical responses that cause certain changes in the hypersensitive lungs. The muscles around the airways tighten, the linings of the airways become swollen, and the glands produce an overabundance of thick mucus, further narrowing the airway passages. The asthmatic breathes in fresh air, but has difficulty expelling old air. As this poor exchange becomes more marked, the severity of the attack grows. The old air contains carbon dioxide, and the buildup of this gas in the body can be very dangerous.

How common is asthma?

According to *The American Asthma Report* (1989), there are 10 to 15 million Americans suffering from asthma, and that number is rising, particularly among the young. The National Center for Health Statistics indicates that the prevalence of asthma increased 58 percent in six- to eleven-year-old children during the 1970s. In the 1980s, among children eighteen and under experiencing chronic respiratory problems, the percentage diagnosed as having asthma rose from 33 percent to 52 percent. Approximately 7 percent of American children have asthma (the number is higher in boys, urban children, and black children). Nearly three out of every four school nurses have reported an increase in the number of asthmatic children in recent years.

Increased prevalence of asthma among urban children and blacks may be related to overcrowding with increased exposure to mites (unproven).

Increased rates of death from asthma have been highest among blacks and have been associated with poverty at least in some communities. This suggests one of the causes of increasing rates of death from asthma has been inadequacies of medical care due to financial barriers, including lack of insurance.

Hospitalization among children younger than fifteen years old was found to have increased 145 percent between 1975 and 1984; asthma is the leading cause of pediatric hospitalization today. One out of every five children with asthma was hospitalized in 1988, compared with 5 percent of asthmatic adults. And emergency room visit statistics are even worse. Half of the children with asthma went to the emergency room for an asthma attack in 1988; 30 percent had multiple visits.

The number of children with chronic asthma is increasing not only in the United States but in England, Scandinavia, New Zealand, Australia, and Africa. We are not alone—this problem is worldwide! Studies currently underway are examining several possible reasons for this increase. Is it due to better diagnosis and reporting? More exposure to environmental and industrial pollutants and allergens? Synthetic preservatives used in foods and drugs? Other factors yet unknown?

The American Asthma Report states, "Regardless of the exact prevalence, childhood asthma ranks as one of the most common causes of ill health and not only creates a myriad of physical and emotional problems for the child but an emotional and financial burden on the family."

What is a bronchial spasm?

The best description of a bronchial spasm I have heard was given by Dr. Robert Scanlon of Georgetown Hospital. He said there are two sets of nerves in the lungs. Whenever you cough you experience a spasm caused by one set of nerves. When a spasm occurs, a message is sent to your brain and then down to your adrenal glands to send up adrenaline to the second set of nerves. The "second team" coats the first set of nerves with this adrenaline, and the lungs are brought back into balance, ending the spasm. In an asthmatic, not enough of the adrenaline gets to the first set of nerves, or their response to the adrenaline is inadequate, and the lungs remain in spasm. If you want to find out what a bronchial spasm feels like, try breathing through a straw.

What are the most common triggers of asthma?

Some of the triggers are allergies, respiratory infections, exercise, environmental irritants, emotional stress, temperature changes, and drugs.

Allergies. An asthmatic may be allergic to a substance through breathing, touching, or ingesting it. Common allergies via touching or breathing are to animals; pollens from trees, plants, or flowers; mold spores; insect parts; house dust; dust mites often found in mattresses and box springs. Substances that can trigger asthma are found in chemicals in furniture and floor waxes, spray disinfectants, and deodorants; many household cleaners; paints; cosmetics; and sulfites (a preservative often sprayed on fruits and vegetables to keep them looking fresh, and used in some restaurant salad bars as well as in some drugs). Food allergies include allergies to nuts, legumes (beans, peas, peanuts, peanut butter, soy beans, and lima beans), milk and dairy products, eggs, shellfish, citrus juices, some wheats, barley, corn—the list can seem endless. Fortunately some food allergies are outgrown, making mealtimes in grown-up years a lot more pleasant.

Respiratory infections. Colds, flu, and other viruses can trigger an attack. In some children, asthma is often complicated by pneumonia. Coughing is frequently an indication of a pending attack, and is soon recognized as the first sign of trouble ahead.

Exercise-induced asthma. Engaging in sports or other strenuous activity often triggers asthma attacks. Often these episodes occur only in certain types of weather or during seasonal weather changes. Other asthmatics experience exercise-induced asthma in all types of weather. New medications (see chapter 4) have proven very effective for exercise-induced asthma.

Environmental irritants and industrial pollution. Exhaust fumes from cars, buses, and trucks, as well as smoke from burning leaves, cigarettes, cigars, and fireplaces, are very common triggers. Smog and fog can also cause trouble. Scientists still have much to learn about the toll that pollutants take in terms of asthma and many other diseases.

Emotional stress. Although emotions seldom cause asthma attacks, they can intensify episodes. When a child is having difficulty breathing, he can become very fearful, adding to his problems by hyperventilating. Relaxation exercises (see chapter 11) are extremely helpful. Sometimes prolonged laughter or coughing can cause spasms that lead to asthma attacks. The fear and anxiety of anticipating an attack can sometimes bring one on. If the child's asthma is not well managed, and he misses many days from school and falls behind his friends in school work, it can have a devastating effect on his self-esteem, and eventually worsen the attack.

Changes in temperature. A drop or rise in barometric pressure, rain, humidity, or extremely cold air can cause asthma.

Drugs. Drugs are often implicated in asthma attacks. Aspirin has long been known as a trigger for some adults, and is now a suspected cause for attacks in children. Therefore, it is wise to use products that do not contain aspirin (acetylsalicylic acid). Drugs containing the yellow dye tartrazine, often used in the treatment of depression, can be very harmful to asthmatics. Normally harmless drugs can have a reverse reaction when taken in combination with asthma medication. Never give your child *any* medication without checking with your doctor first.

*   *   *

These lists demonstrate there are hundreds of triggers that can cause the chemical reaction in the lungs
that results in an asthma attack. Some parents are
lucky enough to pinpoint the triggers, and are able to
avoid many of them. In our three children, *all* of these
things were triggers at some time or another. In some
instances, we could avoid them, but most of the time
we could not. Some of the triggers bothered our children more in one season than another. We had to
work out a good medical regime for each child, and
constantly refine and readjust it as we went along.

Are all asthma attacks life threatening?

No. Asthma attacks can range from very mild to very
severe. Some children may never need a shot of adrenaline or hospitalization. They are treated successfully
at home and experience little discomfort due to their
asthma. Most asthma attacks are not life threatening,
even if they require some medical intervention. However, without proper management and good medical
supervision, the threat of a very serious attack always
exists.

Will my child outgrow asthma?

Some children do "outgrow" asthma, or at least reach
a point where it no longer interferes with their lives.
There are no guarantees, though. Some children who

have an early onset of asthma have a remarkable lessening of episodes after the age of six, because the peripheral airways increase in size after age five. In my children, and in many of the asthmatic children I observed in the pediatric office where I worked, asthma persisted through puberty and into the early teenage years. After the age of fifteen or sixteen the lungs seem to be less hypersensitive than before. It is very important that children approach these years with their asthma under control, as this control seems vital to the lessening of the episodes. Proper treatment and management of the disease will ensure healthy lungs, and your child will be able to enjoy a normal life when his asthma attacks subside. Without this good control other lung diseases may develop.

If there is a lapse of several years between asthma attacks, don't assume that the old medications should be put to use again. Consult a doctor for a new diagnosis. If recent history is any indication, you will probably find that the course of treatment has been improved by newly developed medication and approaches.

Sad to say, asthma can return in the adult years to someone who thought he had outgrown it. Again, proper control in the early years will make a difference later, both in terms of conditioning and discipline in controlling the disease.

Does asthma cause permanent lung damage?

Asthma is a disease causing reversible airway obstruction. *Reversible* is the operative word here. As long as a child receives prompt medical treatment for his asthma, his lungs return to normal condition when the attack is broken. With aggressive medical treatment, the episodes will be further apart and less severe, and some cases will be prevented entirely. Children who do not receive medical supervision or who do not comply with their medical treatment can develop permanent problems. Pulmonary function tests and the use of flowmeters (see chapter 4) are very useful in measuring the efficiency of the lungs.

Is asthma inherited?

It can be. The findings are that if there is a family history of asthma, the risk of a child developing asthma is greater, which does not mean that your child will develop asthma automatically. My brother-in-law comes from an asthmatic family, and married a woman with asthma. They have three grown children, none of whom has suffered from asthma. My father had chronic bronchitis, eczema, and food allergies as a child. He most likely had asthma, but in those days asthma was often misdiagnosed. He was said to have "weak lungs," and developed severe ragweed allergies as an adult. I never developed asthma. My two sisters and their children and grandchildren do not have asthma. My husband, Gary, had asthma when he was young. Children from asthmatic backgrounds inherit the tendency, but not necessarily the disease.

Do children ever die from asthma?

When Pamela and David were diagnosed as asthmatics, we were told it was a serious disease, but few deaths resulted from it. In the last few decades, the number of deaths from asthma has increased in many countries. Dr. R. Michael Sly, Melissa's specialist, is an outstanding expert concerning mortality due to asthma in children. In a recent article[*] he stated that deaths reported due to asthma from 1979 to 1984 had increased each year and there have been further increases each year since then. Some of the increase may be due to a more precise diagnosis and reporting, and an increase in air pollution. Several factors have been recognized that might help identify children who could be in a high-risk category:

1. Early onset of asthma, particularly in the first year of life.
2. Many wheezing episodes that result in hospitalization.
3. Oral or inhaled corticosteroid dependence.
4. Excessive use of beta-adrenergic aerosols.
5. Labile (unstable) asthma with "morning dipping" diurnal airway obstruction.
6. Noncompliant patients with severe asthma.

The number of deaths due to asthma still remains small in relation to the number of children who have

---

[*] R. Michael Sly, M.D., "Mortality from asthma, 1979–1984," in The Journal of Allergy and Clinical Immunology, Vol. 2, 5:1.

the disease; however, these findings do emphasize the importance of understanding the nature of asthma and the necessity of good daily management.

In two reports published on October 3, 1990, by the Journal of the American Medical Association (JAMA), there is an analysis of the startling increase in the rate of asthma occurring in children in the United States in the last decade. The alarming results indicate that more children are being hospitalized for severe asthma, and that deaths from asthma are also on the increase. These reports indicate aggressive medical treatment is vital to good control of the disease.

> *After a near fatal attack when I was in seventh grade, I began to fear that I would die from asthma. No one had ever explained exactly what had happened to me during that attack, and I couldn't remember. I started to feel safer in the hospital than at home. I would be monitored there around the clock.*
>
> —MELISSA

Should we move to another climate?

Many families who have moved from one area to another in the hopes of helping their asthmatic child have found that the child experienced only temporary improvement. After several months or years, many of these children developed allergies and sensitivities to things found in the new surroundings. Meanwhile, the family has torn up roots and often made financial sacrifices. The emotional impact of relocation results in a further strain on the whole family. Over the years, people who have moved to more barren climates to avoid asthma have missed the trees, grass, and flowers they left behind—so they have planted them. Now they have transplanted not only themselves but the very things that cause asthma. Moving is not the answer. Aggressive medical treatment is much more effective.

Why is dehydration a problem with asthmatics?

The Greek word for *panting* is the origin for the word *asthma*. The short, shallow breathing, or panting, so characteristic of an asthma attack causes dehydration, or evaporation, of body fluids. In addition, the overproduction of mucus can cause vomiting, as can some of the medications used to control the attack. Excessive vomiting causes dehydration. Thus, it is important to encourage the child to drink plenty of liquids. Liquids should be at room temperature, as hot or cold drinks can cause further problems in some children. It may take some cajoling, since a child in the midst of an asthma attack has little enthusiasm for drinking anything. Success at home might avoid a trip to the hospital, though, because the intravenous treatment necessary for rehydration can be given only in the hospital.

When should we call the doctor?
How do I evaluate an attack?

Some attacks are slow in developing; some develop very rapidly. If your child has taken his asthma medication and he is still wheezing, call your doctor. The earlier you notify the doctor of an impending attack, the better the chance of reversing it. Notice the area around the Adam's apple in the neck. Is it pulling in and out? This movement is an indication of distress. Look at the rib cage above the abdomen. If it is pulling in and out, that is, *retracting*, air is caught in this area due to the difficulty in expelling old air. Is the child's breathing very rapid? Is he whiney? Pale? Is there a tinge of "blueness" around his mouth? Is he tired from the effort it takes to breathe? Don't rely on the wheezing sound alone to gauge the seriousness of an attack; when the air exchange deteriorates, no wheezing sound can be heard. With a few simple lessons your doctor can teach you how to evaluate an attack with an inexpensive stethoscope and a flowmeter to assess airway obstruction. *Remember:* At the first sign of attack call your doctor, and continue to keep him advised if the attack continues.

How effective are asthma medications?

When Pamela and David were small, there were relatively few medications. Asthma was a crisis intervention disease. It seemed we were always waiting for the next attack to occur. Today the new medications (see chapter 4) are very effective. They allow aggressive treatment that can both control and prevent attacks. Don't be upset if at certain times more medications are added to your child's regime. It is not a step backward. Instead, it reflects your doctor's capacity to reevaluate the child's treatment plan, and to seek the most effective combination of medications to control the disease. Never add *any* medications yourself without first checking with your doctor.

What is status asthmaticus?

When your child is seen at the doctor's office or emergency room of the hospital because he is having an attack that his regular medications have not controlled, he will be given injections of epinephrine (Adrenaline) or terbutaline, along with breathing treatments. If he does not rapidly improve after several shots, he will be admitted to the hospital to receive intravenous (IV) medications. The admission diagnosis will be *status asthmaticus*, which is just a fancy Latin way to say *asthma*.

What is the most important thing I can do to help my child?

The most important thing parents can do for their asthmatic child is to have a clear understanding of the disease. Learn the physical nature of asthma, exactly what is happening to the respiratory system when he is having a wheezing episode. Know the names of all his medications, their purposes, the amounts to be taken (usually measured in milligrams), and the schedule for how often they are taken. Choose a doctor who is a specialist in asthma, and with whom you can establish good communication. When you've done these things, you will become an expert in the management of your child's asthma, and you will be confident of your ability to handle any and all of the many faces of this disease. Most important, you will no longer be fearful, and your positive attitude will provide the most significant factor in overcoming your child's disease.

3

❖   ❖   ❖

Choosing Your Child's Doctor

" A sthma is a very common complaint and
although it is fre-
quently mild, it is occasionally disastrously severe. In
some instances it fluctuates rapidly within hours so
that the patients are often accused of malingering.
The fickleness of this commonplace disorder, together
with our inability to offer a definitive cure, often ap-
pears to create a negative response in many good doctors, irritating some and frightening others; such
sentiments are all too easily transmitted to our patients and mistrust ensues."[*]

Lessons are best learned through experience, and

---

[*] *From the Foreword by M. Turner-Warwick, in* Asthma, *by Clark and
Godfry, W. B. Saunders Company, Philadelphia, PA, 1977.*

our family's experiences with doctors over the years have dictated my philosophy in working with them.

WHO'S IN CHARGE?

Pamela wheezed every day for more than two years as an infant. I remember when she would attempt to run across the room as a toddler, stopping to lean against a chair, desperately trying to breathe more easily—shoulders hunched, coughing, wheezing loudly, her little heart beating so rapidly.

Our pediatrician had a huge practice, run on a first-come, first-served basis. On one of our visits Pamela and I took our usual seat in the crowded waiting room. The nurse, to my surprise, called us immediately into a treatment room. She had noticed a bluish tinge around Pamela's mouth.

The doctor examined her quickly, told me she was in heart failure and would probably not last the night, and to get her to the hospital immediately. Since help from a rescue squad was not a phone call away then as it is today, I drove to the hospital unsteadily, clutched Pamela to my chest like a football, and raced past the reception desk and to the pediatric ward before anyone could stop me.

The end of that story was happier than the beginning. Quick treatment brought down the size of Pamela's enlarged heart in less than twenty-four hours, and no permanent damage was done. We found that Pamela had hit a crisis due to a mixture of medications. A prescription for codeine to calm a severe cough had interacted with her regular asthma medications and caused heart failure. She was being treated by both her pediatrician and a specialist at the time, and although both were interested in her best welfare, schedules and time constraints meant that they didn't always check with each other on prescription of medication.

So much for the prognosis that "no one dies from asthma." Our baby had come much too close. It became clear to Gary and me that it was up to us to know the medications she was on, the amounts and schedules for taking them, and their desired effects (and undesired side effects).

Even more important, it was up to us to decide who her primary physician would be—who would give a "yea" or "nay" on the mixture of medicines and the types of treatment. We chose her specialist. Although she saw her local pediatrician for other infections and ailments not related to asthma, the specialist would always be consulted about medications for any and all problems.

Lesson number one: Who's in charge? We are. You are. The parent must take primary responsibility for knowing the disease and making many of the choices involved in fighting against it.

FOLLOW YOUR INSTINCTS

My second lesson was learned outside the realm of asthma, but taught me, nevertheless, something about helping an allergic child. Both Pamela and

David were born in an era when breast-feeding was out of favor, and formula substitutes were encouraged. Pamela developed milk allergies within a few months, and none of the various formulas we tried were successful. We eventually turned to goat's milk that our milkman delivered at an astronomical cost.

When David was born, we hoped to avoid similar problems by giving him a new soybean formula. He gained weight, and seemed to do well, except for persistent gastrointestinal problems. For the first three months of his life he was unable to have a bowel movement without assistance, which included not only various medications, but daily physical massage as well. Our doctor finally sent us to a proctologist. The examination was quite painful for David, and when it was over we were told he probably had a condition called Hirschsprung's disease. The proctologist told us it would take fifteen minutes to describe this disease, and he was too busy to explain it. He instructed us to take David directly to the hospital for x-rays, and to arrange to have tissues removed from his large intestine for analysis.

Instead we went directly to the library. The symptoms of Hirschsprung's disease as listed in the medical textbooks did not fit David's symptoms. We decided to get a second opinion, and asked Pamela's asthma specialist, who told us she had never encountered Hirschsprung's disease in a child that young. She advised us to discontinue the soy formula, and to switch to a combination of evaporated milk and boiled water. David has never had any gastrointestinal difficulties since that day. His problem was the soybean formula!

I discovered through this experience that it was up to me to use my common sense. I knew my child. I suspected he didn't have Hirschsprung's disease, and I was not going to submit him to the procedures the proctologist had recommended—not without a second opinion.

Lesson number two: If there is any doubt in your mind about the accuracy of a diagnosis or prescribed course of treatment, follow your instinct and get a second opinion.

BE PART OF THE TEAM

When Melissa started to have very severe asthma attacks in recent years, I was struck by the dramatic change from our earlier experiences with her. Before, when we brought her to the hospital with breathing difficulties, intravenous medication would solve the problem quickly. Now, there were times when we took her with an attack that was not extreme—not getting worse, but just not getting better. She would be given the usual course of treatment, and within a half hour her whole respiratory system would start to shut down. Dangerous levels of carbon dioxide would build up in her blood—a life-threatening condition.

I mentioned to her pediatricians and to various doctors in the hospital that I thought there must be something specific precipitating these crises. It seemed to me that when she got the epinephrine, which was supposed to lessen the attack, suddenly she was much worse than when she first came in for treatment. Could the epinephrine be causing the problem?

They didn't listen. They talked more about what should be done the next time Melissa came in with a severe attack—how to get her to the intensive care unit immediately. When I was put in touch with Dr. Sly, her new specialist, I mentioned my theory to him. I told him I knew nothing about pharmacology, but my observations told me that something wasn't working the way it should.

He mulled it over, and commented that I might just have something. He mentioned that both the epinephrine and Alupent, the drug of choice for follow-up breathing treatments, contained sulfites, which can cause an allergic reaction on their own in a small percentage of the population. Perhaps this treatment was the precipitator. He advised that we try a drug called terbutaline the next time she needed treatment, since it contained no sulfites. We would use forms of it both for the initial and the follow-up medications.

A creative idea, but Dr. Sly was out of town when Melissa headed to the hospital the next time! Both she and I dreaded another hospital visit, but a gorgeous warm fall that brought everyone else joy had developed mold on the leaves and rasping in Melissa's lungs. We couldn't avoid some kind of hospital intervention, with or without Dr. Sly.

When I got to the local hospital, I asked that Melissa be given an immediate shot of terbutaline, and that the pediatric resident be called to confer about continuing treatment. Hackles began to rise. The nurse moved Melissa to another treatment room, making her walk from one area to another, despite her wheezing. The emergency room doctor wanted to know if I was sure I wanted to cause the delay that calling the pediatric resident would demand. And did I know that terbutaline, although it had been accepted by the Food and Drug Administration (FDA), required extra paper work when given to children?

At that point I spoke clearly and forcefully. I wanted the intervention done that I had outlined, and I didn't want to argue, because that kind of tension would only cause apprehension in my child. The staff did respond, and it worked. Melissa's blood gases never built up with carbon dioxide as they had in previous recent attacks, and she was out of the hospital within several days, without having experienced another respiratory shutdown. And the people who had fought me at first now became my strongest supporters. Most of the doctors there now say the treatments that had once given her relief in those earlier months could have caused severe distress.

I was certain the doctors and nurses who had resisted these changes actually wanted the best treatment for Melissa. It was just that they had become committed to a treatment that had worked so well with so many children that they lost sight of Melissa as a unique individual. I did not. When it comes to my child, I'm the expert. I'm the keen observer. My observations are worth noting.

It is too bad that we so often run into an "us" and "them" mentality when we go to a new physician or to an emergency room. If the parents don't know much about asthma, the medical team disregards them totally. If the parents, on the other hand, are knowledgeable, the doctors may get a message that says, "Who are these smart alecks who think they need special treatment?" If you're told, as I was so many times, that "It's not in the literature," remind them that you're writing the literature—you and your child—every day.

Perhaps the best analogy here is one from sports. The doctor is the coach, and the parent is the quarterback. The parent has to read the defenses and know what is going on. When the parents give their report to the doctor about what they have seen and what seems to be happening, the doctor can bring his or her medical expertise into play. Without that combination, the team can't score.

I now have a letter from Dr. Sly stating that terbutaline will be the drug of choice for Melissa in emergency situations. I also know to contact my local pediatricians before taking Melissa to the hospital to ask them to get in touch with the pediatric resident on call, so that he can meet us in the emergency room.

Lesson number three: Make certain that the medical team listens to *you*. Get past your fear of ignorance and embarrassment to guarantee at all costs that your observations will be taken into account.

Putting these and other lessons together, Gary and I have been able to make some tough choices in selecting doctors over the years. When you have a child with a chronic disease, your doctor is as important as a spouse. Choose carefully!

SELECTING THE DOCTOR(S)

Asthma is high on the list of diseases that physicians dread. It's hard to treat; it ties up a treatment room;

it's a 3 A.M. call. With advances in asthma medication, and better understanding of the underlying causes, the outlook for treating the disease has improved dramatically. It's important, though, that you select a doctor who is well versed in the treatment of asthma, one who views the disease as a challenge rather than a nuisance.

You may want to pick a pediatrician who is also a specialist, or you may want to use two doctors—a general pediatrician and a specialist. This latter choice may be especially appropriate if you have had a fine experience with a pediatrician up to the time your child first exhibits asthma symptoms, and you want to stay with that original doctor.

The most important consideration is that you choose a doctor who takes a real interest in your child's condition. In the parlance of the medical profession, a child with asthma is usually called a "wheezer." You want to be sure that your doctor thinks of your child not as a wheezer but as a person who *also* wheezes.

You will need a doctor who will treat asthma aggressively. When you sit down with a prospective doctor to discuss your child's and your family's history, ask him what his expectations are—how he intends to treat the disease. If he talks mostly about crisis management, you've probably got the wrong person. What you're looking for is someone who plans to work with you to control asthma on a continuing basis.

Since there are so many changes and advances in this field of medicine, ask a doctor about recent research pertaining to asthma. Can he cite recent findings and the latest experiments in medicine? How often does he go to medical conferences? Fine updates are offered at the best medical centers throughout the country. (There is a point of diminishing returns to this kind of travel, of course. You want your child's doctor in town and near a phone most of the time so he can be available in emergencies.)

Working With Your Doctor

You, your child, and your doctor are going to have a long-term relationship, one that involves more frequent contact than would be true in a family without asthma. You will be conferring with him a great deal. It is important that you feel comfortable talking to him, expressing any fears, concerns, reservations— anything at all that concerns your child's asthma.

Do you need to check the exact doses and times for medication? Call him.

Do you have some doubts about how well a course of treatment is working? Call him.

Have you noted a marked change for the worse in your child, even in the middle of the night? Call him.

Has your Aunt Millie or Mrs. Johnson down the street told you of a miracle cure that has been in her family for years, or of some drastic danger facing your child that has never been mentioned before? Ask him. Chances are 98 percent that these old wives' tales are misinterpretation of the facts, but it's worth checking out.

It goes without saying that your relationship with your doctor will work best if you consider his schedule and the pressures on his time. Call during his "phone" time whenever possible. Collect questions that don't need answering immediately. Write them down and ask them all during the next office visit.

When you go to the doctor's office, and your child is wheezing, tell the nurse at the front desk that your child is having an asthma attack. You should be put in a treatment room right away. Either the doctor or one of the nurses should listen to the child's chest immediately. If your doctor's office is not run this way automatically, ask to be put in a treatment room and to have the child checked as soon as possible. You will be able to gauge, very quickly, how seriously this office treats a wheezing child.

I would also suggest periodic consultations with your doctor, even when things are going well. If your child is taking medication, that could be every four to six weeks. If good fortune has really rained on you, and your child is off medicine for the time being, once every six months should do it. You will have a more leisurely time to discuss how your child is doing, what happened recently, and how your child is doing without medication.

If your doctor speaks to you in "medicalese"—and most slip into it at one time or another—don't be embarrassed to tell him you don't understand him. Ask for an English translation. You and your doctor can't work as a team if you don't speak the same language.

Changing or Adding Doctors

If your child's asthma is under good control, and is not interfering with his life, then you have the right medical support. However, if he is missing school, having acute attacks and hospitalizations, then you need to reassess your choice of doctors. Although your local doctor may be able to treat a variety of illnesses, he may not be the best physician to handle chronic asthma.

The mark of a really fine doctor is his willingness to tell you when it's time to seek another opinion, a fresh look. That frequently doesn't happen, though. Too many parents are hesitant to ask their pediatricians for a referral to an outstanding specialist in the area. If your child's asthma has been unstable for some time, it is your responsibility to broach the subject with the pediatrician and to seek out a specialist who has chosen to dedicate his or her career to this difficult disease.

Every region of this country has outstanding medical facilities, with eminent physicians on staff. Gary and I are fortunate to have Children's Hospital in the Washington, D.C., area, where experts in pediatric medicine are given the opportunity to do what they do best—practice medicine and research—without the small business preoccupations of a private practice. There is always time for excellent communication between doctor and patient, which results in better understanding and management.

A good local doctor will remain very important in treating your child, and will welcome the advice of a specialist. The expert will evaluate your child and work up a treatment regimen that he will communicate to you and to your local doctor. The sooner your asthmatic child with continuing difficulties is evaluated by an expert, and a course of treatment is started, the closer you are to controlling asthma so it will no longer interfere with your child's life.

One final note. The above advice should not be interpreted as a suggestion that you hop from one doctor to another in search of a magic cure. No one has it. The solution is getting the right combination of medications to help your child. It doesn't happen overnight; the adjustments take place over a period of time. It is up to you to determine whether the refinements in medication are really making a difference after an appropriate waiting period.

WHEN IT'S NOT JUST THE LUNGS THAT HURT . . .

Asthma is a demanding, frustrating, and frightening illness that can strain the emotional fabric of the whole family. Professional counseling is often useful in restoring perspective and making everyday life more manageable. Ask your doctor for advice. Sometimes a family session with him will help. Your family may want more than one session with a professional counselor. Don't be reticent to reach out for the help you need for everyone's mind and soul, not just your child's body.

CHAPTER

4

✿   ✿   ✿

From Gunpowder
to Cromolyn

When my husband, Gary, was a little boy in the 1930s, he swears that one of the medications given to him when he had asthma was a form of gunpowder! He would pour a small amount of powder into the top of a tin, ignite it, and inhale the fumes. The rationale: The smoke would make him cough and bring up mucus.

Another of his medications was a long cigarette, three quarters filter, with powder at the end. He was told to light the cigarette and inhale the smoke, again with the idea of coughing to clear his lungs. The active ingredient in the powder and Asthmador cigarette was stramonium, a weak bronchodilator with activity similar to that of atropine.

Gary remembers many sleepless nights, sitting up

in a straight-backed chair trying to breathe. He particularly remembers missing the 1939 New York World's Fair because of wheezing. Decades ago, life could be particularly difficult and disappointing for a child with asthma. There were few ways to avoid the debilitating nature of a disease that robs its victims of oxygen.

Thank goodness today's medications do a better job of controlling asthma than Gary's gunpowder did. Because of them, he has usually been able to fulfill his promise to himself and his children that they would not miss something that was important to them because of asthma.

FALSE STARTS

When Pamela was small, the drug of choice for asthmatic children was aminophylline suppositories. Aminophylline is a very effective drug when given intravenously during a difficult episode of asthma, but can be quite dangerous when given by suppository because of the erratic rate of absorption. If excessive doses are given, the drug can be toxic and even lethal.

Pamela continued to wheeze daily, and to awaken most nights coughing and choking. Gary would walk her for hours, holding her over his shoulder. Finally our doctor prescribed ipecac, which we gave her every night for months. The theory was that the core of the mucus plug causing her worst difficulties with asthma was in the stomach, and that to rid her of it we had to make her vomit. In the last few years there has been a great deal of publicity about ipecac because teenagers and young women with anorexia and bulimia misuse it to lose weight. It can be very injurious to the stomach, and should not be used with any frequency, certainly not every night. I am disturbed, too, when I think of the physical and emotional discomfort Pamela suffered when she was made to vomit night after night.

By the time David came along, several oral theophylline drugs were available. One was called Tedral. It acted as a depressant in our children. If there is one thing worse than a wheezing child, it's an unhappy wheezing child!

Another drug we tried was called Marax. At the 1964 Olympics a swimmer, Rick Demont, had to return his Olympic medal because he failed to inform the judges that he was taking Marax to control his asthma. Marax has a stimulant called ephedrine in it. Not only did Rick Demont stop taking Marax but so did we.

If your child has just been diagnosed as asthmatic, feel fortunate that it has happened in the 1990s. In the last few decades so much has been learned about asthma, and many new and better medications have been developed and refined. It is likely that your child's asthma attacks can be controlled or even prevented. It's just a matter of finding the right doctor and receiving the necessary combination of medications to meet the child's needs.

HOW THE SYSTEM WORKS

In order to understand the purpose and usefulness of asthma medications, it is important to know how the respiratory system works, and what changes take place during an attack.

We breathe in air through the nose or mouth, into the larynx (throat), and through the trachea (windpipe), which branches into two tubes called bronchi. One of these bronchi enters each lung and splits into many branches called bronchioles. At the end of these branches are air sacs called alveoli. The oxygen we breathe goes from these air sacs into the blood, and is pumped through the body. The air sacs also remove carbon dioxide from blood. Carbon dioxide is the waste product of the air we breathe in, and we eliminate it by exhaling. The smooth muscles of the airway passages control the flow of air into the air sacs. During an asthma attack, these smooth muscles tighten around the airway passages; the linings of the passages become swollen and filled with blood cells, and the mucus glands in the lining tissue produce thick, sticky substances that further plug the airways. Breathing becomes forced, and air going through the narrowed passages causes vibrations, thus creating the wheezing sound. The lungs can become overinflated due to the trapped air behind the airway passages. Good air exchange—the breathing in of fresh air and the exhaling of old air—breaks down, and carbon dioxide builds up in the body.

Asthma medications are used to prevent or reverse these changes in the body. The most common medications used for treating asthmatics are theophylline, beta-agonist drugs, steroids, and cromolyn sodium. Let's look at each category of drug to identify what it can and cannot do.

THEOPHYLLINE DRUGS

Theophylline drugs are bronchodilators. They relax the smooth muscles of the airway passages, and relieve airway obstruction.

Examples: Theo-Dur, Slo-bid, Slo-Phyllin, Somophyllin, Theolair, Quibron.

Purpose: Theophylline drugs are used mainly as maintenance therapy to help control and prevent symptoms of chronic asthma, to control exercise-induced asthma, and to help control intermittent acute episodes.

Side effects: Most common side effects are overactivity, nervousness, upset stomach, nausea, vomiting, and headache. When erythromycin is being taken for infection, theophylline stays in the system longer and the doctor may reduce the dosage of theophylline.

Notes: The dose of theophylline is determined by the child's weight and age, and the dose should never be increased without the doctor's approval. It is important to have regular follow-up visits with the doctor to be sure a growing child is receiving the proper dose.

Theophylline has been an important drug for all our children. Each of them has taken it daily for asthma as he or she grew up. Pamela and David have not required any asthma medication in years. Melissa still uses theophylline daily, and theophylline levels are very important in her case. When Melissa has a viral infection, she metabolizes theophylline differently. Her usual blood level is doubled, meaning the theophylline dose must be reduced. At the first sign of flu-like symptoms—nausea, vomiting, headache—we go immediately to the doctor's office to have her theophylline level measured. Other things can cause a change in the way the body metabolizes theophylline, including several other drugs (cimetidine, ranitidine, oral contraceptives, allopurinol, norfloxacin, ciprofloxacin can increase theophylline blood levels, while active or passive smoking, phenobarbital, phenytoin, rifampicin, carbamazepine, and nifedipine can decrease theophylline blood levels). If your child is taking it routinely, have the theophylline level measured at your doctor's office or the hospital every few months. A small amount of blood is taken from the child and tested to be sure the dose is within the therapeutic range.

Be sure that the dosage is taken as scheduled, since the object is to obtain a blood level that enables a sufficient amount of the drug to reach the lungs. This goal is achieved by taking the medication at regular intervals. At the first indication of wheezing, the theophylline medication should be started. It should be continued until three or four days after the symptoms have disappeared. If the child takes the medication too infrequently, it is ineffective. If he takes it too frequently, it can become toxic. Directions should be followed exactly.

BETA-AGONIST DRUGS

Beta-agonist drugs are also bronchodilators. They relax the bronchial smooth muscles, relieve airway obstruction, and may inhibit the release of histamine and other chemicals caused by allergies. They can be taken by mouth or inhaler.

Examples: By mouth—metaproterenol (Alupent, Metaprel); albuterol (Proventil, Ventolin); terbutaline (Bricanyl, Brethine). By mist or inhaler— albuterol (Proventil, Ventolin); metaproterenol (Alupent, Metaprel); terbutaline (Brethaire), bitolterol (Tornalate), pirbuterol (Maxair), isoetharine (Bronkosol). Albuterol is available also as a powder in capsules (Ventoline Rotacaps) for inhalation after perforation of the capsules in a special inhalation device (Rotahaler).

Purpose: Beta-agonist drugs taken orally are often prescribed if the child cannot tolerate theophylline. They are sometimes an add-on to theophylline to make it more effective. They prevent the symptoms of chronic asthma, control exercise-induced asthma, and help control intermittent acute episodes.

Beta-agonist drugs taken by inhaler provide relief of symptoms more quickly than those taken by mouth. They relieve exercise-induced asthma, help control many inhaled triggers, reverse mild wheezing episodes, relieve sudden-onset episodes, give relief while theophylline drugs build up, help control breakthrough (wheezing despite the use of other medications) episodes while the child is on theophylline, open airways before cromolyn use, relax bronchial smooth muscles, and relieve airway obstruction.

Side effects: The most common side effects of beta-agonist drugs taken by mouth can be rapid heartbeat, pounding in the chest, shakiness, nausea, vomiting, nervousness, and headache.

The side effects of beta-agonist drugs taken by inhaler are minimal if the inhaler is used properly, because the drug goes right to the lungs rather than through the entire system.

Notes: Unfortunately, children often use inhalers as if they were breath fresheners. They squirt them into their mouths and do not get the full effect of the medication. They use inhalers *much* too frequently. At *every* visit the doctor should have the child demonstrate how he uses the inhaler, and should go over the correct procedure with the child:

1. Shake the inhaler.
2. Exhale the old air from the lungs.
3. Activate (push) inhaler while breathing medication in slowly.
4. Hold medication in lungs five to ten seconds.
5. Exhale slowly.
6. Wait two minutes and repeat first five steps.

The proper use of the inhaler can take thirty seconds for each intake. Some children do only a quick spray because they are embarrassed by being seen using the device. Convince your child of the importance of using the inhaler correctly. Otherwise the medication will not take full effect and the child will feel the need to use the inhaler too frequently. Your doctor will tell you how many puffs per day the child can take. Do not exceed that amount! As with all medications for asthma, compliance with your doctor's directions as to amounts and frequency is vital. If the drugs are improperly used, they will not produce the full effect. Use of a special inhalation chamber such as

Aerochamber, InspirEase, or Inhal-Aid, facilitates delivery of medication to the lungs for those children unable to synchronize inhalation with activation of the inhaler.

When my children were in elementary school, I asked the nurse or clinic aid to notify me if one of them needed to use the inhaler, which resided in the nurse's office, more than once during the school day, so I could assess the problem. Had he just participated in strenuous physical exercise? Had he just come in from a cold or windy recess? Or was he wheezing continuously? If he was having difficulty getting through the day, he probably needed more than the inhaler, and his appearance in the clinic was an indication of that.

ANTICHOLINERGIC DRUGS

Ipratropium bromide (Atrovent) is a bronchodilator that acts in a different way from beta agonists. It is one of a group of anticholinergic drugs which include atropine and stramonium, the active agent in the type of smoke my husband inhaled as a youth to control wheezing. These drugs work by inhibiting impulses carried by the vagus nerve that tend to constrict the airways. Ipratropium is prescribed most often for treatment of chronic bronchitis, but it can also improve lung function in some people with asthma. Improvement in lung function after inhalation of both ipratropium and a beta agonist is sometimes better than after either drug alone. It is not a substitute for a beta agonist because ipratropium has a slower onset of action, but the effect may last longer than that of a beta agonist. It may be beneficial for asthmatic patients whose asthma is triggered often by emotional factors or irritants.

STEROIDS (CORTICOSTEROIDS)

Steroids suppress the adrenal glands but also reduce swelling of airway linings, limit production of mucus, and allow beta-agonist drugs to be more effective. They are very powerful drugs with undesirable side effects, and their use must be closely monitored.

Examples: By mouth—prednisone (pill or liquid); Medrol (pill); Prelone (liquid); prednisolone (liquid). By inhaler—Azmacort, Vanceril, Beclovent.

Purpose: Steroids are used when an attack is not responding to other medications, and a short-term use of steroids can reverse the attack and allow the other medications to become effective. Steroids are used in the long-term management of severe asthma that is unresponsive to other medications used by themselves.

Steroids taken by inhaler are mainly for prevention of attacks. When a child is having an episode, the inhaled steroid does not provide a large enough dose for the management of the emergency, and the medication cannot get through the narrowed passages; therefore, it should not be used for treatment during a wheezing episode. The benefit of inhaled steroids, as with beta-agonist drugs, is that the medication goes directly to the lungs rather than throughout the body's system.

Side effects: Some of the side effects of steroid drugs can be growth inhibition, susceptibility to infections, water retention, acne, facial puffiness, weight gain, stretch marks and thinning of skin, cataract formation, increase in body hair, headache, increase in urination, and high blood pressure. Although it is important to be aware of possible side effects, with proper management many can be avoided. Some side effects, such as facial puffiness, water retention, acne, and weight gain, disappear when medication is discontinued. Use of a chamber (Aerochamber, InspirEase, Inhal-Aid) can help prevent side effects from much of that portion of the dose that otherwise would have been left in the mouth.

Notes: The use of steroids need not be alarming to parents or the child. The object of their use is to prevent a serious episode that could be life-threatening. Much has been learned about their effects on the system; with proper dosage, side effects are controllable. When used in long-term management, alternate-day low doses are given. The medication is taken in the morning when natural steroid production by the body is highest. By giving the drug on alternate days, the side effects are reduced.

When steroids are no longer necessary, the child is taken off them slowly, in decreasing dosages, in order to permit recovery from any adrenal suppression (the adrenal glands, which have not functioned at top level during the long-term use of steroids, are given a chance to take over again). Steroids are never used unless they are absolutely necessary to control severe attacks. Properly used, their benefit far exceeds the risk of side effects. Pulmonary function tests and flow-meter rates (see page 56) should be done routinely to be sure that airway obstruction is reversed.

CROMOLYN SODIUM

Cromolyn sodium is one of the most important advances in the treatment of asthma. It prevents the release of chemicals by the body in reaction to allergy-causing substances, and thus inhibits bronchospasm induced by allergies. By coating the lungs with cromolyn sodium, the medication makes them less hyperreactive, and allergens, such as animals and cold air, do not cause the lungs to react. Cromolyn has proved effective in 65 percent to 80 percent of asthmatic children in preventing or reducing the severity of asthmatic episodes. Many children have been able to cut back or eliminate other medications.

Examples: Intal (by Spinhaler [see explanation below], nebulizer, or inhaler).

Purpose: Cromolyn by Spinhaler is used by inserting a powder-filled capsule into the Spinhaler (a special inhaler that permits perforation of the capsule and inhalation of the powder) and then inhaling. It is used three or four times a day to prevent asthma episodes. It is also effective in preventing exercise-induced asthma when it is used before exercise. The cromolyn solution comes in ampules, and is taken in mist form by using a small mask and tubing connected to a nebulizer driven by a compressor. It is usually used three or four times per day, as prescribed by the doctor. Cromolyn by regular inhaler is now available, as well.

Side effects: The most common side effects are throat irritation, unpleasant taste of the powder, coughing, dizziness, and rare allergic response to cromolyn. Sometimes patients become unresponsive to cromolyn after periods of good control, due to worsening of the asthma.

Notes: When Melissa tried cromolyn by Spinhaler, she found the propeller easy to use, but we saw no improvement. However, when Dr. Sly shifted her to the use of the nebulized solution and the compressor, allowing for more individualization of her dosage, the results were spectacular. Since each child's asthma is different, the dosage and form of medication vary according to the child's special need. Thus, it is important to seek medical support from a physician who has the time and interest to work out the most effective treatment plan for your child.

The most important ingredient in the use of cromolyn is your child's cooperation. Cromolyn is a preventive medication, and must be used every day at prescribed frequency if the medication is to be effective. Cromolyn is not effective during an attack. Often with the relief of symptoms the child stops using his Spinhaler, nebulizer, or inhaler and the asthma episodes return. Eventually the lesson of cause and effect is learned.

PUTTING IT ALL TOGETHER

Melissa, our third child and the one whose severe asthma has lasted longer into her teenage years than her two siblings, serves as a good example of a successful search for the right medications to control asthma.

When she first went to Dr. Sly a few years ago, the medications that had been working for her had lost some of their effectiveness. We needed the analysis only a top specialist could give. He took a medical history that consumed three or four hours in the telling. He took her through allergy tests again, tested for cystic fibrosis again, and methodically ruled out numerous possibilities. Then he readjusted her medications, making what would seem to the layman to be relatively minor changes. He knew, though, that these delicate modifications could make the difference for Melissa in controlling her asthma.

Today she takes cromolyn three times a day, using a compressor. She also uses the compressor for breathing treatments with other medications as needed. If she suffers wheezing between cromolyn medications, she takes a premixed Bronkosol breathing treatment that usually controls the episode. These occasional breathing treatments are extremely helpful for acute, sudden-onset attacks. The treatment relaxes the muscles and allows her to control the attack until further intervention can be given as necessary.

The compressor is portable, and runs on electricity. Melissa usually takes it with her when she spends the night at a friend's house. The combined use of cromolyn and the breathing treatments have prevented or controlled many episodes. We have found the compressor essential to the successful management of Melissa's asthma. Your doctor can write a letter to your insurance company explaining the necessity of the compressor for your child's treatment, and it is likely that insurance will pay the major cost of the equipment. Also, many electric companies, upon receipt of a letter from the doctor, will give priority to your neighborhood when restoring lost power. The purpose of these programs is to ensure that customers who depend on electricity to power machinery vital to health are not deprived of service for extended periods. You'll be surprised at how popular it will make you with other families on your block!

CHECKING IT OUT

There are two tests that aid in measuring the progress of your efforts to control your child's asthma on a continuing basis. You'll learn about them as time goes by, and find them useful.

Pulmonary Function Tests

These tests estimate the degree of airway obstruction. The maximum volume of air a child can forcibly exhale in one second is compared with the volume of air when completely expelled. This test is done in your doctor's office, and by comparing the results before and after medication, the doctor can judge the effectiveness of that medication. The child may be asked to run in place, so the results of strenuous exercise can be measured.

Pulmonary function tests also measure the total lung capacity. The results of these tests, done periodically, are important in diagnosing the seriousness of the disease and its progression. They are very valuable in developing a treatment regime.

Peak Flowmeters

Much less complex than pulmonary function test instruments, peak flowmeters are available at low cost for use at home in monitoring lung capacity. The child blows into a plastic device as hard and fast as he can. The meter records how much air he expels. The child does this test three times, and takes the best reading of the three. If the peak flowmeter is used each morning and night, differences in lung capacity can be noted, indicating changes in airway obstruction. Often an impending attack can be anticipated, and medications can be given to forestall the episode. The use of the meter also gives both parents and doctor a good indication of how effective the current medical regimen is. If your child has seasonal asthma, charting his daily lung function at the start of the season will give you and your doctor good information as to when to start medications.

As you can see, we have come a long way from the gunpowder remedy for asthma! So many different medications and methods of taking them are available now. We can provide our children with information, good medical and parental support, and the medications themselves. But we can't wheeze or stop wheezing for them, so it is up to the children to follow the regimen. A small inconvenience for a normal, asthma-free life!

> *What would I say to kids who have asthma today? I'd say "Don't smoke! Be optimistic! Take one day at a time. And never go anywhere without your puffer!"*
>
> *—PAMELA*

ALLERGY SHOTS: WHO NEEDS THEM?

The idea that allergy shots (immunotherapy) are a "cure" for asthma is a widespread myth. Many of the triggers that cause an asthmatic episode are not caused by allergy. Allergy shots are important in reducing sensitivity to specific allergens, such as pollens, molds, and house dust, but their use in the management of asthma is not called for automatically. For Pamela, they were of little use in reducing her symptoms. For David, they were a necessity in controlling his seasonal symptoms. For Melissa, they were a trigger that caused her to wheeze.

Pamela's asthma was almost uncontrollable, requiring many hospitalizations. The medications available were limited, and allergy shots were one of our few options. Today, shots are not given during an attack. Pamela wheezed every day, all through her series of allergy shots. Perhaps they were of help in reducing some of her hypersensitivity to seemingly everything under the sun, but no dramatic results were noticeable. After several years her specialist and the local pediatricians agreed the shots should be discontinued.

David's asthma was triggered mainly by infection, exercise, and seasonal changes. He received allergy shots for about six years. They not only reduced his seasonal symptoms, but he developed fewer infections. The shots undoubtedly contributed dramatically to the reversal of his allergies to pollen, grasses, trees, and molds, permitting him to pursue his chosen field of horticulture.

Melissa has been skin tested, and allergy shots have been attempted three times over a thirteen-year period. However, she could not tolerate even the small amount of extract of the allergy-causing substances, due to the extreme hypersensitivity of her lungs. The same day she received a shot, she would have an asthmatic episode. In her case, the shots themselves brought on an attack.

How They Work, When They Work

When a child is allergic to certain allergens, the body produces a protein, called an IgE antibody, against each particular allergen. The IgE antibodies attach themselves to basophils, which are a type of white blood cell, or mast cells, which are tissue cells found mostly in the linings of the respiratory tract, gastrointestinal tract, and skin. When the allergens are encountered, the mast cells then release chemicals called mediators which can produce the typical asthmatic changes in the lungs.

When allergy is suspected as one of the causes of your child's asthma, your doctor will skin test your child to identify which allergens are responsible. A diluted amount of each of the most common allergens found in your locale is either injected under the skin or scratched on your child's arm or back. A small red area will develop, called a wheal. The size of the wheal will signify the degree of allergic reaction. A serum is made up of diluted extract from the offending allergens, and the child begins a series of allergy shots. The series begins with small doses once or twice a week, and continues with larger doses given less frequently. The purpose of these shots is to build up the child's tolerance to the allergens. The process can take several years.

The success of allergy shots is dependent on the child's receiving the shots at regularly scheduled intervals. If the child does not come regularly for his shots, the gradual increase in dosage cannot take place.

After receiving his shot, the child should be prepared to wait in the doctor's office at least twenty minutes for the reaction to that shot to be measured. This measurement is done by noting any redness or irritation at the site of the shot.

FOODS AND ASTHMA

When Pamela and David were born, breast-feeding was discouraged; they were both formula babies. Foods were introduced in the first few months of life, and they developed allergies to milk, soy formulas, and many foods. When we attempted elimination diets, which demanded experimenting with very strict prohibition of a variety of foods, they were almost impossible to follow. Manufacturers did not list all the ingredients on food products, and we had little information on food additives and chemicals found in foods. Suffice to say, both children had very difficult and sickly infancies.

When Melissa was born, we had learned a great deal about both asthma and allergies. I breast-fed her for six months, with no supplemental bottles of formula and no foods. She was our healthiest infant, and has had relatively few infections since birth. Nursing Melissa did not prevent asthma, but it did delay the onset of the disease.

If I were pregnant today, knowing our family history of asthma and allergies, I would start preventive steps immediately. Based on extensive reading on allergy prevention, I would breast-feed my child. For the last three months of my pregnancy, and certainly while nursing my child, I would avoid eating foods that are most commonly associated with allergy. These foods include milk, eggs, peanuts, nuts, wheat, soy, citrus drinks, and fruit.

I would work very closely with my doctor in adding vitamin or calcium supplements to my diet. I would nurse my children for at least six months, without supplemental bottles or any food. A recent study in Scotland showed that babies breast-fed early in life are one third as likely to develop gastrointestinal infections as bottle-fed babies. If necessity demanded supplemental bottles, I might try a soy-based infant formula (Nutramigen, Pregestimil), but even soy milk can cause allergies. Experts say that perhaps a better choice is hydrolyzed, or partially digested, cow milk.

My children would receive no untreated cow milk, corn, wheat, citrus, beans, or peas for the first year of life, and no eggs, chocolate, fish, peanuts, or other nuts until they were at least two. Eggs, milk, peanuts, soy, wheat, and fish account for 90 percent of food sensitivity in children. I would add cow milk to their diets very slowly, and watch for reactions carefully. The protein and lactose in cow milk have been shown to be a major allergy problem. If my child were allergic to cow milk, I would become a food label junkie, looking carefully for such terms as whey, casein, NA caseinate, and cheese to warn me away from foods containing cow milk products.

I would add foods to my child's diet one at a time, three or four days apart, so that I could observe any reactions. I would keep a diary of those observations. I would interview my prospective pediatrician, in-

form him of our history, and be sure he was support-
ive and knowledgeable about current research into
aggressive prevention of asthma and allergy. These
steps are no guarantee that allergies to food will not
develop, but I firmly believe they are worth taking.

Food Detectives

All that is fine, you say, but how does a parent predict
allergies that might show up during the first few
months and years of a child's life, well before asthma
has reared its ugly head? One way is to remember
your own history. A child has only a 10 percent likelihood of developing a reaction to food if neither of his
parents has an allergic disease. He is 70 percent to 80
percent likely to do so if both parents suffer from
allergies. Clues other than asthma often show up early
in the game, skin rashes, diarrhea, and vomiting fore-
most among them.

Food allergies and intolerances can develop at any
time. Frequently, if the foods are eliminated from the
diet for six months to two years, children outgrow
many of them. An *allergy* to food means that the child
cannot eat any of that food without a reaction. If a
child has an *intolerance* to certain foods, it means
those foods can only be tolerated in small amounts.
Sometimes the adverse reaction occurs immediately,
sometimes not for many hours after the food has been
ingested. A common reaction is in the form of hives
(urticaria)—red, raised welts—or swelling (edema). If
your child develops hives or swelling, contact your
doctor right away. The child may be swelling inter-

nally as well as externally. Your doctor will probably prescribe an antihistamine such as Benadryl or Atarax. However, if the reaction is severe, the child may require adrenaline.

What can you do for your child if allergies show up after infancy? Even today, with better labeling of food products, elimination diets are not easy, but they're worth trying. You'll probably do better with an expert allergist or nutritionist guiding you than with attempts at self-diagnosis, but several books are listed in the Appendix that will give you the details on food allergies, their symptoms, and elimination diets that address them.

Don't be discouraged or frustrated with elimination diets. One of the hardest things to do is to break bad eating habits. Consider this an opportunity to start your child off with good ones!

There is another consideration related to food that has little to do with allergies but could have something to do with asthma—weight. Logic says that a child who carries extra weight around on a constant basis could be adding to his asthma troubles, especially if that weight discourages him from exercising. As children grow, increased weight is often followed by a spurt of growth in height. If that doesn't happen with your child, and his weight begins to exceed the average ratio of height to weight shown on your doctor's chart, perhaps some subtle diet changes are in order.

At present there are no skin tests that identify conclusively adverse reactions to food or medications that can prevent those reactions from happening. Perhaps these will be among the future marvels added to the giant steps that have already been taken in the treatment of allergies.

When Pamela was a Brownie Scout, I was one of the leaders of her troop. David would usually attend the meetings with us, and participate in whatever craft project we undertook. One week we decided to make birdfeeders, and one of the ingredients was peanut butter. We knew David was allergic to it—he even hated the smell of it. He applied the peanut butter to his birdfeeder with a knife. Within minutes, huge red hives appeared all over his body, and his lips and eyes started to swell. We went directly from the meeting to the emergency room of our local hospital, where he received a shot of adrenaline. Just touching the stuff caused a severe reaction. Both Melissa and David are still allergic to peanut butter and to peanuts; they are careful never to eat anything made with peanut butter or cooked in peanut oil. People allergic to peanuts may tolerate peanut oil.

David has been a vegetarian for the last three years. Not only is he a wonderful cook but he feels better in every way since he changed his dietary habits. Vegetarianism is not for everyone, but a better understanding of good nutrition is.

This chapter on medications, allergy shots, and diets once again points out how vital the roles of parent and child are in the daily management of asthma. There is no quick "cure," just many different methods of control. The more information you have about the causes of the disease and the available treatments for it, the better that control will be.

5

✿ ✿ ✿

Going to the Hospital

FAMILY TIES

It is strange (or perhaps not so strange) that people in Third World countries have a better understanding of the price of separation and the benefit of continuity of family life than we do. Often, when a patient is hospitalized in a "primitive" culture, family members accompany the patient to the hospital and camp close by. They prepare the patient's food and serve him in whatever small ways the hospital will allow. They maintain the family connection. Psychological and physical separations are avoided. Family life goes on as it should.

Americans handle hospital stays differently. Our hospitals are highly specialized, antiseptic places. Everyone on the staff has a specific job to do. The family seems to get in the way more often than not.

For the parents of a sick child, especially an asthmatic child whose condition has demanded very active treatment up to the time of hospitalization, this experience can be numbing. From the time the attack started, to the first medications, to the treatments at home, to the decision to go to the doctor's office, to the final drive to the hospital, these parents have been the child's link to health and survival.

Now their role has been usurped by medical experts, and the anxieties appear that the earlier activity concealed.

First Things First . . .

That sense of separation and fear need not overwhelm you. The first thing to remember is that your child has been admitted to the hospital because there is usually no other choice: It is the best place for him to be.

A stay in the hospital is frequently called for in the treatment of chronic asthma. The medications the child has been taking by mouth, the mist treatments with the home compressor, or the adrenaline administered in the doctor's office—none of these has been fully effective in breaking the attack and bringing breathing back to normal. Intravenous medication is needed, and that's only available in the hospital.

As difficult as this experience is, keep in mind that it is nothing really unusual for an asthmatic, and that your child will be headed home in just two or three days. Undeniably there will be feelings of panic the first time you take your child to the hospital. I know what it's like. You're suddenly caught in a freeze frame. Your life stops. Somehow there you are on an ice floe, isolated from the everyday world outside the hospital doors. It's important, though, to control that panic as quickly as possible.

> *I remember spending every Halloween in the hospital, because I was so allergic to the leaves falling then. But I never looked forward to Halloween with fear. My parents never let me be pessimistic—always optimistic.*
>
> *—PAMELA*

You may be fortunate enough, as our family has been, to be at a hospital with a fine pediatric ward, where the support system is good. Or you may be smart enough, after reading this chapter, to find out in advance where the exemplary pediatric wards in your area are, and ask your doctor about the likelihood of using one of them in case your child's asthma requires hospitalization. However, a fine hospital is not the only factor—perhaps not even the most important factor—in your child's well-being during this critical period.

Your positive attitude and your pleasant rapport with the staff are absolutely vital now. So vital, in fact, that a recent study indicated that the ultimate health of a child with severe asthma—whether he lives or dies—may depend to some degree on whether his family has a good or bad relationship with his medical caregivers.

And take heart. It all gets easier and more routine as time goes by.

Little Things Mean a Lot

As you walk into the room your child has been assigned to, you have an opportunity to make a choice that may make a real difference in the days ahead—the location of his bed. If you have your choice of locations in a room with two beds, skip the bed next to the window with the lovely view of meadows and trees or the parking lot outside. Instead, take the bed on the inside, next to the bathroom. Within a day or two your child is going to be well enough to get up and go to the bathroom, still connected to the intravenous tubing. If he's in the bed by the window, the view doesn't help much when he has to get up and drag the intravenous stand behind him like an unwilling pet, hospital gown flapping open in the rear. It's easier all the way around to be a few feet from the bathroom door.

Just the Facts, Ma'am

Once you're settled, the traffic will start through your child's room. If you're lucky enough to be in a teaching hospital, the traffic gets heavier. Three or four people, perhaps even more, will come in asking for a medical history. What happened? Why is the child there? What is the background of health problems, current attack, medications, and so forth?

You may usually consider yourself an organized, analytical person. Don't count on that now. You've been concentrating on a child with increasing symptoms of asthma emergency. You've been too busy to really notice each step the doctor has taken in treating your child. So use a simple solution to the medical history dilemma. When the doctor tells you your child is going to be admitted to the hospital, ask him for three or four photocopies of recent treatment given in his office, which you've probably visited several times over the last few days. Now when the questions are asked in the hospital, you can hand a sheet to the inquirer, knowing that the important points are covered as best as possible.

As the hospital stay continues, you'll want to write down what happens there. Chart the daily medications your child takes, and the last hour taken. These include treatment in the emergency room. One more careful eye on the routine is helpful to the staff in the long run.

May I Help?

As you settle into the hospital routine, start observing how the staff functions. See what you can do to help lessen the burden of some of the nurses' duties without getting in their way.

Our first daughter was hospitalized for the first time twenty-odd years ago. Pediatric wards weren't like those today, with semiprivate or private rooms. They had real *wards*, with plastic partitions between cribs. Visiting was allowed for only a couple of hours in the day, perhaps one hour at night. It was very difficult. We spent too much time wishing we were there when we couldn't be.

Pamela was in an oxygen tent, and she and I felt our separation acutely. I asked the nurse if I could sit on a stool and just put my hand into the oxygen tent and hold hers. I made absolutely no demands on the staff, and made certain the other children could not see me. I just sat quietly and held Pamela's hand. And I found that in performing that function—comforting my child and staying out of everyone else's way—I helped the staff, too.

Part of the help you can provide comes from giving your child the impression that this visit to the hospital is the most natural thing in the world. "Yes, here we are in the hospital. Okay, now what shall we do? What would you like?"

What I usually do is go straight to the hospital from the doctor's office. Don't go home first for bedclothes and personal items. There is time for that later. Of course, you may be at the hospital already if your child has had an emergency that needed immediate attention (see "In an Emergency" at the end of this chapter). But the usual sequence of events finds you first at the doctor's office, with a hospital visit to follow because the acute attack hasn't broken.

Stick around for a while after your child is admitted, because there is blood work to be done and intravenous tubes to be put in. No child wants to face that without you. You can help, too, by suggesting—

as they put the IV tubing in—that they check the doctor's orders to find out what blood work is called for and take the blood samples at that time. There is no reason for the child to suffer the trauma of several needles half an hour apart when one session will do.

Then get your child acquainted with his surroundings. Show him where the bathroom is. Find out if you can wash his face. Make an inventory of the room; show him where the equipment is—ice water, tissues, television. Tell him the plastic cups, hand lotion, tissues, and so forth will be his to take home. You, or your insurance company, will pay enough for them that you might as well give him the little pleasures of ownership right from the start.

Very often hospitals have VCRs. If that's the case, sign up for one. There may be a waiting list, but soon you'll be able to tell your child, "Guess what! We're going to see your favorite movie tonight." Most children like to see the same thing over and over again. Whatever it is, *Superman,* or *Mary Poppins,* or *Saturday Night Fever,* he'll have something to look forward to.

Touches of Home

Once your child starts to feel a little better (it may be within an hour or not until the end of the day) you'll have a little time to note the things he needs, and then head home to get them. Bring his pajamas and slippers, toothbrush, and a treasured possession, such as an allergy-free stuffed animal, Barbie doll, or truck. Don't make the hospital into a playroom, however.

Get things that give the child some comfort and have some use. Bring playing cards if a card game will keep his mind off his breathing, or a board game for two. Books that he wants to read or that you can read to him will make the stay more enjoyable. Is the child interested in music? One of your best investments may be a little radio with earphones.

Don't Call Us . . .

This hospital stay may be short, but you'll still need all your strength and ingenuity to keep your child occupied and as happy as possible. Your first priority must be that child, not a lot of concerned relatives and friends.

When you get calls in the hospital from worried relatives and neighbors, remember the child hears every word you say. Watch the length and frequency of your phone calls. A million conversations in which you relate every little detail that brought you to the hospital can be very damaging, because in the telling and retelling things are always exaggerated. Tell the truth, but avoid heavy drama. The best way to handle it might be, "Yes, Susie has had an attack. We just couldn't seem to break it, so we decided we'd come to the hospital. We should be out in a couple of days."

If grandparents and aunts and uncles start arriving from all over the country, then you not only have the child to worry about but you've got guests as well. You're better off to discourage visits from relatives unless you're certain their presence will be a genuine help to you and your child. If grandmother's visit will perk your child up and give you a few minutes' respite, encourage her to drop in. Otherwise tell adult friends and relatives you'll get in touch with them when your child is home from the hospital, and you hope they'll visit at home after the hospital stay.

Try, no matter what your anxiety level is, to bring theirs down. It will help you *and* your child. Remember that asthma is the kind of disorder in which emotions can play a great part. Anxiety only intensifies an attack, so you don't want to be overly anxious or solicitous. As long as you sound positive, as long as your spirits are up, then everyone else's will be too. It is especially important because asthma is not a broken leg, an appendix operation, or a similar one-time thing. You may be back quite a few times. Establish right away that this hospital visit is not an unusual or scary thing but a normal, beneficial treatment for asthma.

How about visits from your child's friends? A few, but not too many, will probably be best. Remember that, depending on the age of your child, he's probably not particularly anxious to have the whole world come over to see him with his intravenous mechanisms and too-short hospital gown. Our family has been fortunate in having enough friends who care about our children to stop in every so often for just a few minutes.

If the child is over eight, he'll be anxious to make and get phone calls. Let him. Friends who hear that your child is in the hospital may think he is grievously ill. If he can pick up the phone and establish contact with them again, everybody's mind will be set at ease. He'll find out what went on in school that day, and his friends will know he is doing fine. It often helps stop a lot of exaggerated gossip that goes along with hospitalization.

> I remember one of my best friends called me when she heard I was in the hospital, and she was hysterical. She was afraid I would die. None of my friends had ever said that to me before, and it really startled me. After I comforted her and tried to convince her I would be fine, I had a long talk with my parents and doctor. I needed their comfort and assurance that I would be fine. I explained my fears and confusion. They told me I wouldn't die and that I alone could control my asthma.
>
> —MELISSA

What about giving presents? It's nice when a few of your friends remember the child and send something over, but you really don't want to start that to any great extent, because your child may be hospitalized enough times to try a friend's patience and budget in the future. Your child's roommate, experiencing his first and only hospitalization, may receive all kinds of flowers and plants and presents. You certainly don't want the flowers and plants, because they may stimulate allergies. And your child will soon realize that gifts cannot be expected on a frequent basis.

All of this advice about visits and phone calls and presents adds up to a very important premise. You don't want the child to become a prima donna. You'd be surprised how fast a helpless youngster can turn into a churlish complainer if you give him the slightest encouragement. Don't let it happen.

Snack Time

When your child is feeling better, it's guaranteed he'll start to get hungry. He'll want an ice pop, some orange or grape juice, some kind of snack. On the floor of most pediatric hospitals are refrigerators containing these goodies. Find out where one is, ask permission, and then whenever possible get snacks for him when he asks, rather than bothering the staff. If you've got a finicky eater on your hands, the hospital may allow you to bring favorite snacks or juice from home.

GETTING QUESTIONS ANSWERED

You'll have dozens of questions to ask as the hospital stay proceeds. What's going on? When can you expect the medication to take effect? What can your child eat? The nurses may be closest to you, but it's not their job to answer these questions. It's your doctor's. Your relationship with your doctor should be comfortable enough to allow you to ask *anything* about the treatments.

You may have noticed that doctors don't sit by the phone waiting for you to call to ask questions. You can get your answers, though, if you plan carefully. If the doctor can't speak to you at the time you call, find out when he can call back. Be there at the time the nurse says he will call you. Write down your questions so you won't forget something important.

If you prefer talking to your doctor face-to-face, find out when he makes hospital rounds. It's usually at the same time every day. Park yourself in the hospital at that time, and be in your child's room when the doctor comes to check him. If you need to ask a lot of questions, walk in the hall with him after the examination and ask them there. After you finish your discussion with him, come back and tell the child what the doctor told you (or as much as you think he can understand) so he doesn't feel there's something being kept from him.

Find out what the child wants to ask, too. If he has questions, have him ask the doctor directly. If your child has entered the hospital via a visit directly to the emergency room, without a stop at his doctor's office, it's especially important to make certain your doctor stops by the room as soon as possible to talk to you and answer questions.

Others on the staff can also be helpful in answering questions. The intern and the resident will probably introduce themselves to you. You can call for the pediatric resident to come and answer specific questions any time you're in the hospital. Remember, though, that the rapport you build up with the staff is dependent to a great degree on whether you ask your questions as a team member rather than as a potential enemy.

Often, as I've worked in a doctor's office with young children, I've seen parents react very negatively to the need to draw blood. "Oh-oh," they'll say, "Bobbie's going to be very upset because he had such a *bad* experience in the hospital." Actually, it's probably the parent rather than the child who remembers the experience as a bad one. The parent may have caused a scene about something he didn't understand or because his anxiety level was so high he just overreacted. If something happens in the treatment of the child that you're not pleased with, there are various avenues for correcting it. In a problem with the nursing staff, don't just strike out at the nurse. Find out quietly who the head nurse is for that shift. Speak to her as pleasantly as you can. Explain the situation, and you'll find either there is a simple answer that you were not aware of, or she'll fix the problem for you. You can also talk to the pediatric resident, and of course to your own doctor. Everyone's memories of the hospital stay will be better if you treat problems calmly.

Sleeping In

The question always arises: Should I spend the night in the hospital? It's advisable for one parent to do so if the hospital allows. In our family I have always stayed. My presence allows for the family continuity that is so desirable. If the child has a problem I'm right there, to give the support that only a parent can give.

Being in the hospital is very wearing, but if you ask yourself, "Where do I want to be when my child is ill?" the automatic answer will almost always be, "At his side in the hospital."

Base each parent's time in the hospital on the logic of who is more available, whose personality can handle it best. In our case, Gary visits often and has a very good outlook. But putting him in the hospital for eight to twelve hours at a time is like putting a lion in a cage. So I don't feel the need to say, "I've been here for six hours, so you should be here for the next six hours." Things can't be balanced that nicely. Given all possible choices, this place is not where either of us would choose to spend our time, but we work out a schedule for these few days that best suits us, as individuals, and our child.

If there are other, younger children at home, there are additional considerations. Because asthma is a chronic disorder, and you're probably going to be in the hospital a number of times, it won't be easy to keep calling on neighbors for emergency help. Careful scheduling is in order. If there are two parents available, one gets up with the homebound children and gets them to school in the absence of the other, who has spent the night at the hospital. One makes sure to be home to greet them after school and feed them, hearing about their day, helping them with assignments, while the other goes for an afternoon visit to the hospital. If you're it in a one-parent family, you'll need to do a careful balancing act with the babysitter. You can work anything out—just try to discombobulate as few people and their schedules as possible.

GOING HOME

When your child is released from the hospital, he will be released because he is no longer wheezing. Asthma is a completely reversible disease, which means that the lungs go back to their normal condition and there is no damage done to them.

Our practice has always been to get the child back to school the day after release from the hospital. Life goes on. Children have the most wonderful outlook. They want to get on with it. When an adult goes into the hospital, he may live through it once, then over and over again in the retelling of the trauma. When the child feels better, he forgets everything else about his sickness, and throws himself back into his routines quickly . . . if given the chance.

Life is about problem solving. You and your child can consider asthma one more opportunity to learn how to solve problems. He may find if he can deal with this problem early in life, other problems that face him later on become much easier to handle.

It's all in the way you look at it.

IN AN EMERGENCY

Emergency room takes on a quite different meaning to parents of an asthmatic child. An emergency room will not usually be the site of some fearful crisis for you. Instead, it can serve as an extension of your doctor's office after his hours are over for the day. It's your twenty-four-hour medical facility when traveling. And it's the first place to go when your child is having a severe attack.

Emergency room personnel specialize in crisis intervention. They tend to be impersonal, and to whisper out of hearing distance from the patient and family. Thus, a letter from your doctor is *essential*. This letter should identify your child as asthmatic, and should outline specific treatments most effective for him. It should introduce you as knowledgeable, concerned parents whose observations and experience will be helpful to your child's treatment.

When you arrive at the emergency room, ask to speak to the doctor in charge. Introduce yourself, and give him your letter. It will ensure that your child gets the right medication and dosage, and will confirm your status as a participant in discussions and decisions.

If your child develops problems after your doctor's office is closed, call him anyway. The answering service will track him down, and after-hours calls are expected by all good physicians. He may be able to suggest additional treatments you can give at home, or he may advise you to go to the emergency room. Ask him to notify the hospital that you are coming, and if the hospital has a pediatric department, have him request that the pediatric resident meet you in the emergency room. If your doctor has given you photocopies of recent treatments (see page 36), take them along.

●●

I can't remember the details. Oh, I remember the hospital and the oxygen tent, but I've pushed the rest away because it was painful. It represented failure. I pretended it didn't exist. When you're younger, you're more resilient. You forget the painful stuff.

—*PAMELA*

One of the bad things about having an asthmatic child in your family is the local emergency room personnel will probably get to know you pretty well. It's also one of the good things in a situation where quick action and mutual confidence are critical to good care. If the doctors and nurses know you and your child, and vice versa, familiarity may breed relaxation and confidence.

Present your letter whenever you need to stop in an emergency room when your family is traveling. In the unlikely event that this letter does not secure proper treatment, remember your doctor is just a phone call away. He will quickly help you clear up any misinterpretations with the emergency room staff. Don't be intimidated; you know your child's requirements better than anyone else, and your doctor will back you up.

If your child has a sudden, acute attack, or if his ongoing attack intensifies, take him to the emergency room immediately. Don't let the episode become more severe by delaying needed treatment. If possible, call your doctor's answering service, have them advise him of the situation, and ask him to call the hospital to alert the appropriate personnel. Going to the emergency room right away may prevent a real emergency.

Treatment given in the emergency room depends on the severity of the episode. Perhaps one or two shots of epinephrine (adrenaline) or terbutaline, and breathing treatments with albuterol, Alupent, Bronkosol, or terbutaline will reverse the attack. Sometimes a shot of Sus-Phrine (epinephrine in solution) is given. It is a longer-acting adrenaline. Medication administered intravenously may be given over several hours in the emergency room. Blood will be drawn to rule out infection, determine the theophylline level, and monitor blood gases. If the attack is not satisfactorily reversed, the child will be admitted to the hospital for a few days.

Once in the hospital, his usual course of treatment will include corticosteroids, aminophylline, and hydrating liquids given intravenously. Drugs administered this way have a more certain and rapid access to the vascular system than those given orally. Theophylline levels and blood gases will be monitored. Oxygen by face mask or nasal prongs will be given, as will regular breathing treatments. As the child's condition improves, usually in a day or two, intravenous medications will be discontinued, oral medications will be started, and the child will be released.

We have visited many emergency rooms up and down the eastern seaboard in the course of our children's disease. After an afternoon or day at the beach, it was not unusual to stop at the local hospital with Pamela and David wheezing in unison. Frequently the emergency staff was more upset than we were. We would reassure them that it was a familiar song. We tried to bring a sense of perspective and humor along with us, and the majority of our visits were positive ones.

6

❂ ❂ ❂

Day by Day

One of the most frustrating things about asthma is the sense of losing control over what is happening to your child and your family. While doctors can give you help in handling crises, what is preferable is to anticipate problems and get a little ahead of the game. This chapter offers a variety of ways to gain more control—things you can do, on your own, to stay out of a crisis mode.

DEAR DIARY . . .

Asthma is a capricious disease, striking suddenly when you least expect it. Detecting the triggers would tax the powers of Sherlock Holmes. To develop your own detecting powers, do what Holmes did: *Keep a journal.* Collect all the data surrounding the attack for clues as to its cause.

Weather

Note the weather conditions on the day of the attack, and try to remember what they were for the several days preceding it. Was it unusually hot or cold? Warm days, cool nights? Was it windy? Were windows open? Did the barometric pressure drop suddenly? Was it raining or very dry? What was the season of the year?

Activities

Chart your child's activities for the week preceding the wheezing. Had his social life been more active than usual? Had he been engaged in strenuous exercise or sports? Did he have less sleep than he usually requires? Was he outdoors for extended periods in the snow, rain, wind, or hot summer sun? What was happening at school—did a pet come for a visit to his classroom?

Physical Symptoms

Try to remember and jot down any symptoms, no matter how slight, of a cold or a sore throat. Have you noticed any nasal congestion or drainage? Did he cough occasionally? Did he clear his throat frequently? Was he irritable or did he seem to tire easily? Did he seem pale? Were there darkish circles under his eyes? Was there any sneezing, loss of appetite, stomach pain, wheezing between medication doses?

Medication

Did your child miss any scheduled doses of medications prior to his attack? Sometimes a child's asthma seems so well controlled that he becomes lax in taking medications, and wheezing develops. If your child takes medication on an as-needed basis, how soon did you start his medication at the onset of this attack? The usual caution parents exercise about not giving their children any drugs until they're absolutely certain drugs are needed doesn't work here. In all the years I worked for a group of pediatricians, I never saw an asthma attack caused by giving medication too early. I witnessed many serious attacks, though, because medications were not given soon enough. Soon enough means *at the first sign* of possible trouble, when a dose of medicine may control or prevent the attack from developing without any further medical intervention.

Did you notify your doctor if your child experienced wheezing that broke through the control of regular medications? How soon did you call him? Write down what procedures he recommended, and how effective they were.

Home Environment

Write down any changes in the household cleaning products you have used in the week or so before the attack. Any new floor or furniture waxes, laundry soaps, or fabric softeners? Did you change your furnace or humidifier filters frequently enough? Did you use any insect sprays or room deodorizers? Did a visitor bring tobacco smoke into the house, or a gift of fresh flowers? Have you changed to a new perfume, or tried new lotions (hand creams, face creams, sun lotions, etc.)? Have you painted the house, or spray painted outdoor furniture?

Foods

If your child has food allergies, have you read carefully each label to check ingredients in the foods you're purchasing? Have you prepared food differently? Our children could not tolerate fried foods, or food cooked on a charcoal grill. Have you combined foods in new ways? For example, Pamela had no trouble with tomato sauce, unless it was combined with eggplant, which would cause a full-blown asthma attack. Has your child been eating at a friend's or relative's home lately? What was served?

This journal will be invaluable in the search for triggers and warning signs. Read over the information you have collected concerning each episode. You will discover common threads and clues that will enable you to avoid certain triggers. You will become sensitive to the first warning indications and start needed medication immediately. You will know what weather conditions cause an attack, and give medication to *prevent* episodes.

And a final reminder: Once you become an expert detective, become an expert paramedic as well. Keep your child on his medicine for several days even if his wheezing stops, to be absolutely certain his lungs have stabilized.

COMFORT CONTROL

The classic asthma attack occurs after the child has been lying flat and sleeping for a few hours. It is hard to breathe in this position, since mucus often clogs the airways. Normal beds cannot be adjusted to provide an angle for the head and shoulders to be raised slightly, but you can accomplish the same thing by putting pillows *under* the mattress. (It provides a gradual rise; the child is less likely to slip down in the way he would if pillows were piled in back of his head on top of the mattress.) This position allows for easier movement of the diaphragm in the abdominal area, and thus easier breathing.

During the winter season you may notice your child experiences a slight soreness in his throat in the mornings, or occasional nose bleeds, or nasal congestion. These symptoms are an indication of dryness in the house caused by your heating system. Such dryness irritates the membranes in the nose and throat, and can trigger asthma. You need more moisture in the house, or at least in the child's room. Sometimes a good humidifier added to your furnace will alleviate the problem, or you might consider a small room humidifier. Don't overuse, however. High humidity favors growth of mites and fungi. Check with your doctor. If he agrees that a room humidifier (which will cost less than a whole-house system) is appropriate, be sure to change filters frequently and follow cleaning instructions carefully.

In the summer months you will have the reverse problem if you live in an area with high humidity. Soggy moist air favors growth of fungi that can trigger asthma attacks. A damp basement may require a dehumidifier to prevent growth of fungi.

Air conditioning is a must for asthmatic children. However, don't turn the thermostat so low that the difference between indoor and outdoor temperatures is too dramatic. Going from one extreme to another causes its own problems. Keep the room or house comfortable—about 74 degrees Fahrenheit—and encourage your child to spend a good part of each day in this atmosphere. It is easily done when children are small. As they grow older, let them invite friends to share a Monopoly game or some other activity that will keep them from feeling imprisoned in their own home or room. Sometimes an air-conditioned movie is an inviting treat. If your car is not air-conditioned, though, avoid trips on very hot days if possible.

If a swimming pool is available to you, it is a good place to spend part of a very hot, humid day. Water is a good "cleanser" for a child's breathing system. Swimming (see chapter 11) is a wonderful activity for asthmatics, but, as with all activities, moderation is the watchword.

In the winter, you may find that once a hard freeze hits your area, your child's asthma improves markedly. The freeze kills many of the asthma-producing triggers. However, cold air can create other problems. Often your child will leave the house in the morning asthma-free. Fifteen minutes later you receive a call from the school to come pick him up because he's wheezing. What happened? The walk to school or to the bus stop in the cold air triggered an attack. You can help avoid this problem by providing him with a long muffler or scarf. The logo of a favorite sports team or college on the scarf can make it worth wearing. He should cover his mouth and nose loosely with the scarf, and he should try to breathe through his nose. The scarf will filter and warm the air before he breathes it in, and he will be able to tolerate it much better.

If your child is not eligible for bus transportation to school, and you cannot drive him there, arrange an appointment with the principal. Explain your weather-related problems, give the principal a letter from your doctor confirming what you explain, and ask permission for your child to board the bus at the stop nearest your house. It will cut down on his exposure to the elements, and with his trusty scarf in place, many of the episodes caused by cold air will be eliminated. Your doctor may direct your child to take several puffs from his inhaler about a half hour before walking to the bus, which is often very effective in controlling problems.

All children love to play in the snow—it's an essential winter ritual. The asthmatic child is no exception, but care must be taken. Several short exposures outside are preferable to long exposure, accompanied by increasingly wet clothing. When your child is very young, and anxious to build a snowman, have him supervise from the window while you do most of the work. Then bundle him up warmly, scarf in place around his mouth and nose, and let him affix the button eyes and carrot nose and arrange the broom in the snowman's arm. In providing all the finishing touches, he will make the snowman his own. Then a quick ride on the sleigh around the yard should ready him for a return to the house.

As your child grows older you can discuss with him the weather conditions that cause episodes. Have him come up with activity plans that accommodate the limitations to exposure. If he plays a major role in framing these plans, he is more likely to comply with them. A few short periods of skating and sledding are preferable to none, and he will enjoy them much more if he isn't wheezing.

When choosing clothing for your child, be sure that you don't buy garments to which he is allergic. Down-filled jackets and wool material should be avoided. Stay away from down-filled comforters and materials that produce lint, like chenille. Thinsulate linings do the trick nicely for jackets and coats, and comforters filled with manmade fibers will keep him warm, and cost less too.

That Uncomfortable, Embarrassing Visit

"Why does my child always wheeze at grandmother's or Lucy's house?" Some children cannot tolerate older homes. It has nothing to do with current house-cleaning procedures, just the accumulation of years of dust and dirt (see chapter 7 on environment). Your child may be fine during short visits, but wheezing starts when he spends the night, or after a few days. Find out if there is a bedroom that can be allergy-proofed (see chapter 7) before he visits.

Do your relatives or friends have pets? Is there a fragrance worn by grandmother that your child can't tolerate? Were the floors and furniture newly waxed in anticipation of your visit? Are there houseplants? Is the heating system humidified? Perhaps you can bring a small portable unit with you. Does anyone in the household smoke? Cigar, pipe, and cigarette smoke cause many attacks, and the air is polluted long after the offending substances are extinguished.

Is the climate where your relatives live much colder or hotter than what your child is accustomed to? It might be wise to plan visits during times of the year when these climatic differences are not too extreme. Do your friends and relatives serve foods different in type and combination than your child is used to? Are cooking odors very pronounced?

Note the differences between your home environment and that of your relatives. Sometimes a few simple changes can make a big difference. If those changes can't be effected, explain your child's adverse reactions tactfully and patiently, and ask them to visit you instead. Avoid making anyone feel responsible or guilty. Another idea: Perhaps you can spend the day with friends and relatives away from both your homes, or sleep at a motel when you visit them.

THE ASTHMATIC COUGH

Dealing with the enigma of the asthmatic cough is like steering a boat around treacherous rocks. The cough helps break up the mucus, keeping it loose and allowing the child to spit it out. However, constant dry coughing can intensify an attack. Your navigation tools are liquids. Drinking plenty of liquids keeps the secretions loose and soothes the throat. Ginger ale, Gatorade, apple juice, Jell-O, clear lukewarm liquids like broth or consommé, decarbonated sodas, and ice pops have been staples at our house. Water didn't happen to be one of our children's favorite beverages, but if your child is willing to drink it, the more the better. If your child is not allergic to lemonade, Kool-Aid, or citrus juices, try them. Fruits work too—grapefruit, oranges, plums, or other juicy fruits can be given in sections every fifteen minutes unless your child is allergic to them.

Keep encouraging small sips of liquids if the child complains of being too full. Provide him with a good choice of beverages, but not with the option to decline them all. If your child cannot tolerate liquids due to vomiting, get in touch with your doctor right away.

If your child is successfully treated for asthma at your doctor's office or at the emergency room and then sent home, the need for liquids continues. After an attack, the lungs are in a "twitchy" condition, which means they are highly susceptible to another attack. Controlling mucus is very important at this time, and probably easier, since the child will be feeling much better and will be ready to drink liquids.

Drinking plenty of liquids should not be a some-time thing, reserved for emergencies. Nutritionists say large doses of water and juices are an essential part of regular diet. If your child is accustomed to such a diet on a daily basis, you will not have to force feed him when he is fighting an asthmatic cough.

THE ACUTE ATTACK

When your child experiences an acute attack with very little warning beforehand, his practiced breath-ing exercises (see chapter 11) may fail him due to his anxiety and fear. Give him the required medication, then stay with him, comforting him calmly, in a soothing place. Rub or massage the back of his neck and shoulders, relaxing the muscles in that area. You will find he often holds his shoulders in a hunched position, which is a natural response that elevates the chest cavity to allow him to inhale more oxygen; how-ever, it can make the shoulders very tense and sore.

Urge him to take short, shallow breaths while con-centrating on slowing down the rapidity of his breath-ing. Count the number of breaths per minute out loud, and constantly congratulate him as his breathing slows. As the medication begins to work, and he feels the tightness in his chest loosen, have him start his breathing exercises. Stay with him. Keep encourag-ing him. Never leave your child alone, at home or in the hospital immediately after an attack. Wait at least twenty to thirty minutes to make certain the episode is over.

It is in treating these quickly developing episodes that we have found the small home compressor so valuable (see chapter 4 on drugs). Administering the premixed medication in mist form, with the use of the mask, is the easiest and quickest way to relieve an acute attack or break up a sudden mucus plug that is clogging the airways. However, if after a short time your child requires another treatment, contact your doctor right away. It is an indication that your child's regular medication is not enough and further treatment is needed.

A young child can become very frightened when the mask necessary for the mist treatment is placed over his nose and mouth. If he is using it for the first time at your doctor's office or in the emergency room, take a few minutes to alleviate his fear. Hold the mask up to your face first, and laugh at how "funny" Mommy or Daddy looks, and what fun it is to play this game. Let him put it on and off his face, and smile and clap your hands at how super he looks. If he has a toy with him, have him place the mask on the toy. When he has the mask in place over his nose and mouth, hold him on your lap, his back against your chest, your arms securely around him. Peek over his shoulder and look at him; be sure he can see your face as you sing him favorite songs, tell him a story, or recite nursery rhymes he enjoys. Try to keep his mind occupied on something other than the mask and apparatus. He will relax, and the mist treatment will be much more effective. The masks are plastic, and since hospitals and doctors' offices use them only once, your child can take the mask home with him. Tell him he can teach his favorite bear how to use it when he gets home.

If your child has more than mild asthma, I really encourage you to invest in a home compressor. The home breathing treatments you will be able to administer represent one of the most important advances in the management of this disease. The cost is between $150 and $170, and most insurance companies will reimburse you for a good part of the cost if your doctor writes a letter saying the compressor is needed. When not in use, the mask and tubing should be stored in a zip-locked plastic bag. After each treatment, wash out the mask with hot, soapy water and rinse it in clear water. Use dish-cleaning soap that does not leave a residue. If you are using the compressor to administer daily medication, you only need to wash the tubing once a week. The mask should always be washed before every treatment, however. After washing, attach tubing to the compressor without the mask and turn on the compressor. The air forced through the tubing will evaporate any moisture.

Be sure to practice the use of your home compressor with your child *before* an attack develops. Occasionally let him try the mask on himself or a toy, so that when he must use it, the mask will be an old friend.

CHARTING YOUR CHILD'S
MEDICATION COURSE

When your child is taking daily medication over a long period of time, it is important to devise a simple method of recording the medication given. This process ensures that the prescribed doses are given, and can prevent double doses given by mistake. Draw up a chart for each medication, listing the days of the week and a month's worth of days. A typical monthly calendar with boxes for each day can be photocopied for this purpose.

If your child takes medication twice a day, then the space under each day is divided into two boxes. Each box has the time when the dose is to be taken. As the dose is taken, the appropriate box is checked. Sometimes small round stickers—a different color for each medication—can be used in place of check marks. They brighten up the display considerably, making it more fun to do and easier to read from a distance.

Keep the chart hanging right above the place where medication is usually administered. When your child is taking additional medication (perhaps an antibiotic or additional asthma medication) along with his regular medications, keep a separate chart next to the regular one(s).

As your child becomes mature enough to administer his own medications, this charting responsibility will become his. Oversee his charting for a period of time, until it becomes second nature to him.

Your Own Private Drugstore

Once your child has been diagnosed as asthmatic, the accumulation of daily and as-needed medications will begin. You will want to keep this growing drugstore in one central location. We keep all the medications pertaining to asthma in a large bread box on the back of the kitchen counter. In front of this box is an index card noting the name, purpose, administration schedule, instruction as to when it is called for, and expiration date of each medication. I check this card every few months to be sure all medication is current and at full potency. I also keep any extra masks, tubing, or other paraphernalia in this box. Knowing exactly where to find needed medication and equipment will save you much anxiety when wheezing develops.

P. S.

And a few more tips . . .

- Always keep plenty of tissues handy and encourage your child to spit out mucus. Swallowing mucus can upset the stomach.
- When cooking, be sure the ventilation fan on the stove is turned on.
- Leaving the dishwasher open in the last drying cycle will provide humidity in the kitchen.
- If your child wants to play a musical instrument, encourage the piano, guitar, or any instrument that gives them a chance to enrich their musical experience *without* requiring excessive, strenuous lung capacity.
- A large golf umbrella attached to the bed or a chair and covered by a sheet makes a fine tent when you want a vaporizer to work more effectively.

7

✿ ✿ ✿

A Healthy Environment

A ROOM OR A CELL?

When asthma is due to allergy, avoidance of substances to which a child is allergic should be the treatment of choice whenever possible. Success in controlling irritants in your home may determine the effectiveness of all the other elements in your child's treatment plan. However, there is sometimes a tendency to go overboard in protecting the home from possible triggers or allergens. A stark, antiseptic, institutional atmosphere is the wrong approach. Use your common sense when creating a livable environment. Your child is an asthmatic—not a monk.

The most important piece of furniture in a young child's room is a rocking chair. There is nothing more soothing or satisfying to a child than being held snugly on the lap of his mother or father, while the voice he loves best reads him a favorite story. The parent also benefits from this warm intimacy. Many, many days we rocked and read away our anxieties in the woods of Christopher Robin, or in the world of Richard Scarry, or in the fantasy of Dr. Seuss.

When our children outgrew lap sitting, our tradition of story reading continued. When David was in third grade, and home with asthma, the novel *Jaws* had just been published. As we are originally from Long Island, and spent many summers near the locale of the story, I knew he would enjoy the book. In fact, he became so fascinated with sharks that he read every article and book about them he could obtain. He not only learned about sharks but he learned how to do research, and how to locate information. He became a devotee of the local library, learning to use the card catalog and computerized index. He even contacted Dr. Eugenie Clark, a noted shark expert at the University of Maryland, who told David he had done such a good job that there was no more published research on sharks to be had.

David graduated from college this year with honors; perhaps that asthma attack long ago had something to do with his success. There are so many ways to provide your child with a good environment, and the lack of dust is just one of them.

Keep it Clean

Unfortunately, dust is a real threat to many asthmatics, and your child's bedroom is the battleground.

Since most children spend a considerable amount of time in this room, thoughtful attention to its contents is in order.

The simple, uncluttered look is what you're after. The walls should be painted, not papered, because papered walls can become mildewed; they hold dust more because they cannot be washed and repainted. Window curtains should be made of a washable material, and laundered often. Avoid upholstered furniture, where dust lurks in ever-increasing quantities, and choose pieces that can be cleaned with a damp cloth and products like Endust rather than furniture polish. The richest source of the house dust mite is carpeting. A plain wooden floor or tile in the bedroom is a must. A few small area rugs might be permitted, but they should be washable, and washed often.

Alternatives when removal of carpet is impossible include periodic treatment of the carpet with Acarosan, which kills the house dust mites, or Allergy Control Solution, which inactivates the mite allergens. Acarosan, produced by Fisons Corporation (makers of cromolyn), is available from local pharmacies without prescription. Allergy Control Solution, a solution of tannic acid, is available from: Allergy Control Products, Inc., 96 Danbury Road, Ridgefield, CT 06877 (1-800-422 DUST). This company also sells allergen-proof encasings for mattresses, box springs, and pillows.

Collections of dolls, stuffed animals, books—any object that can collect dust—should not be kept in the child's room. While it takes some ingenuity under these circumstances to help your child decorate a room that will reflect his personality, it can be done.

Posters and pictures can be hung, and should be damp-wiped frequently.

Particular care should be given to the bed (and yours too, if your child sleeps there often) and bed coverings. The dust mite, which can't be seen with the naked eye, lives on the surface of mattresses. Old mattresses should be discarded. The shed human skin and yeasts found on their dark, semimoist surfaces provide a haven for dust mites. Cover a new mattress with a zippered plastic cover, and tape down the zipper end tightly.

Dacron or polyester-filled pillows should also be encased in zippered plastic covers. Periodically wash down all plastic covers with a damp cloth. The dust mite is killed by very hot temperatures, so pillowcases, sheets, and blankets should be washed in water at 158 degrees Fahrenheit (70 degrees Centigrade).

Try to change sheets and pillowcases often. Ideally, the room should be cleaned thoroughly once a week. Keep closet doors closed, and cover heat vents with cheesecloth to minimize the dust they release. Damp mopping or sweeping floors spreads dust; vacuum once a day instead. Keep your child out of the room for at least one hour after vacuuming.

When the room is receiving a thorough cleaning, windows can be opened to air it out. Then they should be tightly closed to prevent wind-blown dust and pollens from collecting on bed covers. Also, night air is often damp, and the change during spring and fall from warm days to cool nights can often be a trigger. The old adage, "Beware of the night air," is often true.

Wash windows in your child's room monthly, using a cleaner with as little odor as possible. Do not hang venetian blinds—they can get too dusty. Wipe shades with a damp cloth weekly. Dirty clothes should be put in a hamper in the bathroom, not collected in the room.

Constant use of vaporizers can cause mucous membrane irritation, and vaporizers often grow molds. Use one only when specifically ordered by your doctor. When a vaporizer is used, be sure to wash and wipe it dry every day before refilling.

Dust Patrol

Maintaining a bedroom as dust-free as possible for your asthmatic child is relatively simple when the child is very young. Once your child is beyond the toddler age, however, if you don't get his full cooperation, nothing will work to keep his room in acceptable condition.

Go over with your child all the items that are appropriate to keep in his room. Make a list of those objects and where they belong, for example, clock, lamp, radio on shelf; lamp, plastic jewelry case on night table. List the areas where nothing should appear: under the bed, under the dressers. List items acceptable on the closet floor: shoes, soccer ball, tennis racket, Barbie case, miniature car case.

Then have him conduct a monthly dust patrol. He will refer to the list, noting the objects that have collected since his last survey. He then has the responsibility of eliminating the dust catchers he has spotted, which usually means putting things back where they belong. He will soon learn the benefits of replacing items in dresser drawers and closet shelves rather than letting them accumulate around the room.

Praise his patrol skills, and be willing to negotiate exchanges of acceptable display items. Giving him this responsibility makes him very much aware of the hazards of clutter to his health, and cuts way down on the dreaded nagging mother or father syndrome. Having a list of what should be in the room gives him a target and makes his patrol effort much easier. It won't be long before he automatically rejects surrounding himself with possible triggers. He will also be more aware of avoiding triggers outside his room.

As I grew, I learned to read my body's warning signals and to take the appropriate precautions, whether through medication or simply by changing my immediate surroundings to avert a serious attack.

—DAVID

DOING THINGS DIFFERENTLY

Because our children had severe asthma, we had to make dramatic changes throughout the house. In fact, we had to change houses! The history of accumulated dust, animal hair, layers of wallpaper and paint, vintage heating systems, and molds and mildew can make present-day life unbearable for an asthmatic.

Our move to a newly constructed home had immediate positive results. The reduction in asthmatic episodes more than made up for the loss of the older
home's charm. We viewed the move as an opportunity to make other changes: curtains on the windows,
no drapes; synthetic rugs instead of wool, and foam
rubber padding under the rugs.

We have found that fresh-cut flowers and plants, so
often pollen-laden, are best left outdoors. Artificial
Christmas trees have helped keep the holiday season
asthma-free.

No smoking by family or friends in the house or car
is our rule. Recent research has shown that children
of mothers who smoke as little as half a pack of cigarettes a day are twice as likely to have asthma and
four times as likely to need asthma medication as
children of nonsmoking mothers.

Filters on the furnaces are changed each month,
and both furnace and air-conditioning units are pro-
fessionally cleaned before use every year. Many heating and air-conditioning companies offer special
spring and fall cleaning rates, and we take advantage
of these offers. We use the fireplace infrequently, and
clean out the odor-producing residue as soon as possible. After vacuuming the house, the disposable bags
are discarded and the material bag covering is
sprayed with a disinfectant.

Fresh fruits and vegetables are washed off before
they reach their bins or baskets. House painting is
done only in fine weather, when the house can be left
open, and when the children can visit relatives or
friends.

Since leaves contain molds, we discouraged our children from leaf-raking or jumping in piles of fallen leaves. Mowing the grass was not a task for the children with grass allergies.

Mold grows in damp areas: bathrooms, basements, laundry areas. Since molds are a major irritant to many asthmatic children, you should police these areas regularly.

On a problem of a larger scale, the growing concern throughout the nation regarding industrial and environmental pollutants has resulted in regulations with positive results for asthmatics. Emission standards for automobiles and industries and the ban on leaf burning are giant steps forward. These efforts should not diminish.

WHAT *NOT* TO BRING HOME

While awaiting the birth of our first child Pamela, Gary surprised me with Suzie Wong, a Siamese kitten. She was beautiful, fascinating, and entertaining. Both Gary and I adored her instantly. Unfortunately, we were soon to find out that cats, especially Siamese cats, often cause asthmatic attacks. When Pamela was diagnosed as having asthma, we had to find a new home for Suzie. She tried out several families before the transition was finally made, and we vowed never to have another pet.

Many years after Suzie's exit, David desperately wanted a boxer dog. His doctor approved the purchase of an apricot poodle as a compromise. Poodles are reputed to have less allergy-producing dander, but even a little is too much. Cinnamon is still with us, and we love him dearly. However, the reality is that pets and asthma are natural enemies, and don't belong together. If you are wise you will resist the temptation to have one. Once a pet joins your family, giving it up can cause emotional havoc for everyone.

And if you must have a pet, the animal should *never* be allowed in the child's room. When animals go outside, pollen can cling to their hair. Pets should be washed frequently with mild soap with little odor. Do not spray tick or flea powder on your pet—your child might be allergic to that, too. Stay away from using household flea bombs that could cause your child trouble. As the urine of animals is a cause of allergies, cat boxes and bird cages must be changed *every day*. Stay out of pet stores.

To our family, "house beautiful" means a home as free of asthma-producing triggers as possible. Many of the changes we made were fairly simple, but the results in controlling the children's asthma were enormous. Around our house we have a saying: "Never love anything that can't love you back." Dust-producing furnishings and decorations don't stand a chance in that philosophical environment.

CHAPTER

8

❀   ❀   ❀

Letting Others Care

INNOCENT UNTIL PROVEN GUILTY

My career as a working mother started after my children were in school, and since I was working in my own children's doctors' office, I avoided much of the guilt and blame other working mothers encounter. However, it is true that the one common trait all parents of chronically ill children seem to have is *guilt,* and working mothers get a double dose.

Most parents believe that they should be able to protect their children from danger, and what signals danger more clearly than an asthmatic child gasping for breath? We feel guilt when they wheeze, guilt

109

when adrenaline is shot into their arms, and guilt when intravenous needles are attached to frequently collapsing veins. Intellectually we understand the cause and nature of the disease and the need for shots and needles, but emotionally we believe good parents should be able to protect their young from these torturous episodes.

What we do to ourselves is bad enough. We certainly don't need friends, relatives, or even other asthmatic parents echoing these unfair judgments. Working mothers, and especially working single parents, seem to be tasty prey for this kind of abuse. When people advise you to totally rearrange your life, ask them if they would like to move in for a while and pay the bills.

It is vital to realize that personality differences in children and adults are extremely important. No outside advisor can dictate how you live your life. I have known many working mothers and single parents who have had complicated demands from their role as both parents and productive employees, but they have managed them. Traveling is essential for some people; their careers depend on it. It's not easy to juggle all these obligations, but it can be done. Friends and family are often eager to help. Don't feel that you are so essential to the daily life of your child that absolutely nothing else matters. If it doesn't fit your personality, staying home could be the worst thing you could do. Know yourself and how you function best, and then take action to put you and your child into the best situation you can manage.

When I became a working mother, I discovered two things. First, I was a better than average employee because I rarely took off personal time. I saved my vacation and sick days for the times Melissa's illness necessitated my absence. I relished the continuity of a work situation. Second, I was a more relaxed mother. Working allowed me to develop a whole new perspective. I was no longer so totally immersed in my family's problems. I was also better able to understand the juggling of work and home that my husband, Gary, had contended with for years.

Home Care Is Best

The best environment for a child who suffers frequent bouts of asthma is your own home. Let's assume you have taken steps to control the known triggers in your home that might cause an attack. All the medications and other paraphernalia are at hand. This arrangement might cost more than taking your child to a sitter who supervises several children, but it will prevent many unnecessary infections so easily transmitted from one child to another. Remember that a simple cold for most children may result in asthma complications for your own.

Of course, the location of your childcare will be decided by many considerations, and you must weigh all your options. Sometimes it may be necessary to locate your child closer to where you work. If you are lucky enough to have a member of your family with a vested interest in your child agree to care for him or her in your absence, it makes sense to be flexible about location.

Selecting Your Substitute

If your child has severe asthma, or frequent attacks, you might want to ask your doctor about the nurses' registry. It is a central file where nurses looking for specific jobs can be located. Often you can find someone with the right medical background looking for a position in childcare. Sometimes the nurse may bring a child of her own along, which is still preferable to leaving your asthmatic child in a room with many young children.

When interviewing a prospective substitute caregiver, whether she is a nurse or not, be sure you both have the same overall views on parenting. Interview carefully; your child's health, and perhaps his life, depend on it. Be honest about your child's asthma, the suddenness of attacks, the need for a calm response, and the triggers that affect his disease. The following guidelines may help you, both during the interviewing of candidates and the beginning of childcare:

1. Ask any questions that occur to you, as specifically as possible. Some daycare providers are unwilling to take responsibility for an asthmatic. They may be squeamish about the possibility of an attack, or they may be unwilling to administer medicine.

2. If smoke or pets aggravate your child's asthma, you must raise these issues in seeking a caregiver. You may find an otherwise perfect situation, but a poor environment will put your child at risk. Placing him elsewhere will enhance your peace of mind.

3. Once selected, educate your daycare provider well. Asthma symptoms can be frightening, especially

to people who are unaccustomed to them. It is important to be able to differentiate between discomfort and a genuine emergency situation. While you cannot be called for every wheeze, you don't want hesitation when your child's lips are starting to turn blue.

4. Make up a package of written instructions that can be used as a ready reference for fast instructions.

5. If possible, stay home with the new sitter for a day or two. It will help both the sitter and your child accommodate more easily to each other.

6. Have your caregiver meet your doctor. Perhaps he or she can give your caregiver a little background on the disease and your child's particular case.

7. Be sure your substitute has transportation or can utilize yours. Don't leave the stick shift home if your sitter can only drive an automatic. The caregiver should be familiar with the quickest route to the doctor's office and the hospital.

8. There may be times when your provider will have to take your child to the emergency room and meet you there. For this reason, it is imperative that your provider, or anyone who will be responsible for your child for any length of time, have a notarized statement indicating she can authorize medical treatment in your absence. Otherwise your child may have to needlessly wait until you are located before receiving treatment.

9. There may be other times when you can avoid the emergency room if you step in quickly—if it is possible for you to pick up your child when he is in distress, have him treated at your doctor's office, and return him to his childcare location while you return to work. Or it may be that you can arrange to have the sitter drive him to the doctor's office.

10. If your child has a nebulizer at home and your childcare is not in your home, you may want to consider investing in a second one at the daycare provider's location. Otherwise you will have to leave work whenever the nebulizer is needed, or lug it along with the child daily. Depending on the type of unit, it may not be feasible to carry it from one place to another and back each day.

11. It is important to give honest feedback about how well the childcare situation is going. Does your care provider delay giving medication because your child is happily involved in some activity? Does she call you too frequently? Does she let him play outside against your instructions because it's too hard on him to sit at the window and watch the other children play? Do you come to pick him up to find his chest slathered with menthol jelly because she's convinced it will cure his cough? Then speak up! Things may be set right if you make your directions clear and firm. They are sure to deteriorate if you don't.

They Need Me So Badly at the Office!

In homes with two working parents, who stays home (or at the hospital) when your child is really sick? You really have to find your own system. Do what's right for you and your child. I know one couple that would sit together at their child's hospital bedside all night until morning, when it was almost a toss of the coin as to who dragged off to work and who remained. One night they looked at each other and said, "This just isn't working." They pulled out their work calendars, determined who could most easily miss or be late or be half awake at work the next day, and the other headed home to rest up for a more arduous work day. It works fine as long as both working parents take their fair share of overnight duty.

Respite Care

When your child's asthma is unstable, it is unwise for both parents to be out of town on business or vacation. But you, like everyone else, will need a little rest and relaxation now and then. In fact, given the stress that asthma can bring to the whole family at times, you'll need this break more than others.

During those wonderful periods of good control of the disease, plan a few days away for yourself. Both you and your child need the reassurance that your constant presence is not required.

As with regular daycare, the person staying with your child for a period of several days must be competent to handle asthma attacks, which can develop quickly even during periods of control. Choose your substitute carefully, whether you employ someone or use a relative, and then provide complete emergency information to handle any situation in your absence. Don't scare your potential substitute to death with possible worst-case scenarios, but be completely honest about your child's asthma, and the added responsibility it might require.

CHALK IT UP!

One easy way to ensure that needed data will be readily available is to invest in a large writing board. Using a magic marker, list all information *not* subject to frequent change:

Doctor(s)	1.	Name(s)
	2.	Telephone number(s)
	3.	Conditions under which to call, for example, asthma attack
Emergency	1.	Telephone number
Squad	2.	Responses to squad dispatcher's questions
		(a) caller's name
		(b) your home address, including cross streets to pinpoint locale
		(c) your home telephone number
		(d) your child's name and age
		(e) condition under which to call: asthma attack causing difficulty breathing
Medication	1.	Location of labeled medications (next to which will be a schedule charting daily doses and times)
	2.	Instructions for use of compressor, if you have one. (The compressor should be put together and the correct dose of medicine set in it, ready for immediate use.)
Treatment letters	1.	A blanket release letter (much like the one you sign each year for your child's school), allowing treatment by doctor/hospital in your absence. Pick up a printed form from your doctor/hospital, or have your doctor provide you with proper wording for the letter. Be sure to have your signature notarized if required.

> 2. A letter from your doctor detailing most effective emergency treatment for your child (see chapter 4)
> 3. Letters should be placed in a labeled envelope and tacked up near the information board.
>
> *Known allergies* 1. Foods—list
> 2. Medicines—list

Information that *will* change frequently should be entered on the board with chalk, so that adjustments and new information can be made easily:

> *Name of local friend or relative available during your absence:*
> 1. Name
> 2. Address
> 3. Telephone number
>
> *Where you can be reached:*
> 1. Name of location
> 2. Telephone number at that location
> 3. Name of social event or business meeting
> 4. Name of host/hostess or person in charge of event or meeting
>
> *Medications just given:*
> 1. Name of medications taken that day or evening
> 2. Time medication was given
> 3. Dosage given
> 4. Time when next dosage should be given

Compiling all the important answers to emergency questions, and having your "answer board" conveniently placed, will give you and your substitute peace of mind and confidence. Also, you can accept last-minute invitations or spontaneously planned outings—if a sitter is available—knowing that the essential data are hanging on the wall at home.

9

❁   ❁   ❁

Relationships:
Attitudes and Perceptions

SCHOOL: A MATTER
OF EDUCATION

When Pamela, our old-
est, first started
school, it was as mo-
mentous an event for us as it is for all parents. We
filled out all the forms in great detail, including her
history of asthma. It wasn't long before I received a
call from the school, requesting a meeting. When I
arrived, I was presented with another myriad of forms
to sign, releasing the school from any legal responsibility due to her illness. They didn't want her to
participate in outdoor recess or indoor physical education. I discovered through this process that written
information was the wrong way to communicate with

the school; I needed to give them an education in person.

There are so many misconceptions about asthma. The wheezing sound alone can be frightening, and even mild episodes can be perceived as critical emergencies. I realized that a little public relations effort was called for to help clear up the many myths and misunderstandings.

Getting Down to Basics

So the routine started. When the children were in grammar school, I would request a conference with each child's teacher about two weeks into the school year. I would advise her of the child's asthma; explain how certain weather changes and allergies related to it; let her know very few attacks were life-threatening. I had provided the school nurse with emergency medications, and I was a phone call away and could be reached at any time. I gave reassurance that the responsibility for my child's illness would never fall on the teacher. My husband and I knew exactly how to handle any episode, and the child's asthma need not cause her any anxiety.

Once the teacher realized we took it all in stride, and with a certain amount of humor, she was able to view the child as just another student, not a time bomb.

Extracurricular Activities

I also met with the nurse or clinic aide and explained the medications and their usage. If she was unfamiliar with inhalers, I'd demonstrate how to use one. She could then be certain the children used them correctly. I made sure I filled out all the medication forms, and labeled the medications exactly as the school required. I asked her ahead of time to call me if one of the children came to the clinic several times during the day. I could then talk to the child, and determine whether more aggressive treatment was necessary. In most cases the wheezing was caused by a blustery day or strenuous exercise, and additional puffs from the inhaler were all that was needed.

When the children went on field trips I would try to go along as an extra helper. If my child couldn't go into the animal houses at the zoo, for example, we could wander around outside without inconveniencing anyone else. I enjoyed the trips as much as the children, and the teacher appreciated an extra hand. If you and your husband are working and not available, you might want to consider sending your regular caregiver.

Missing the Action

During the periods when recess or physical education might cause difficulties, I would write an excuse for that day. None of our children was restricted from these activities for any extended length of time. All of the children took part in school field days. All three were awarded physical fitness awards during their school years.

When the children were absent from school, it was their responsibility to make up class work and homework. If the school was given twenty-four hours' notice, needed books and assignments could be picked up at the office or guidance center by Gary or myself or one of the child's friends. Most of the missed work could thus be completed before the child returned to school. When Melissa was in seventh grade she was in and out of the hospital many times. She still managed to take an active part on the editorial staff of her junior high school newspaper, and maintained a straight-A average.

An unexpected benefit of the children's asthma has been the close relationships we have built with the staffs of the schools they have attended. We have had excellent cooperation, and have come to know some truly marvelous people.

Light at the End of the Tunnel

While our more intensive involvement was appropriate in elementary school, as the children moved on to middle and high school two things happened. First, they took over much of the responsibility for control of asthma and communication with school personnel themselves. The groundwork had been laid carefully; they knew what arrangements were needed after years of our handling the disease together. They could now comfortably handle these special arrangements themselves.

Second, and most heartening, was the fact that they actually did begin to outgrow the disease. Less attention to its vagaries was needed as each year went by, and their independence from it and from us was easier to come by.

The children knew by then just what our precepts were: that education was the first goal of teacher and students, and that asthma should only get as much attention as needed to keep it from getting in the way of that goal. It was one school lesson they learned well. It made the high school years both fruitful and fun.

FRIENDS: LET THEM PLAY

Over the eight years that I worked in a pediatric office, I gained great satisfaction from helping develop and teach a class for parents of asthmatic children. We also held periodic classes for asthmatic children. The main problems expressed by these children were caused by overprotective parents. They were afraid that asthma and their parents' attitudes made their friends perceive them as "weird." Most children want to conform to the behavior of their peers. They want to be part of the group, not singled out as different or sickly. Developing normal relationships with their friends is as important as food and water to growing children. If parents think of their child as disabled, you can be sure that their friends will, too. Let me give you a few vignettes of specific children and their parents as I observed them during these classes. The names have been changed to protect the innocent!

Suzanne

Suzanne's mother was full of nervous energy. She was intelligent, involved, and intense. Whatever captured her interest was sure to become the most important topic of her conversation. Nothing had ever engaged her zeal as much as Suzanne's asthma. She read every article she could find, spoke with Suzanne's doctor weekly, and energetically set out to overcome her daughter's wheezing.

Suzanne complained of the constant questions coming from her mother. "Do you have an extra sweater? Did you remember to drink six glasses of water? Did you take your medicine? Is your hood tied securely around your head? Did you cough, sneeze, or wheeze since I saw you last?" Not only did Suzanne's mother interrogate her continually but she related the details of Suzanne's illness to almost everyone she met, usually talking in front of Suzanne as if she weren't there.

The real problem became Suzanne's friends. Her mother treated them like co-conspirators, questioning them daily. Did Suzanne put her coat on at recess? Did she run in the wind? Did she taste some forbidden food they had provided? Finally Suzanne found that her friends began to drift away. They somehow felt responsible for Suzanne's occasional asthma attacks. Not knowing how to deal with Suzanne's mother, they stopped dealing with Suzanne.

Tommy

Tommy was confronted by the "taster." His mother was positive that food allergies were the primary cause of Tommy's asthma. She read every label diligently, and served her family only "approved" foods, discouraging any meals outside their home. Pizza, fast-food hamburgers, and snack foods never found their way onto the dinner table. Tommy's siblings did not have asthma, and they resented the restrictions imposed on them.

Tommy was not allowed to participate in school or neighborhood birthday parties where forbidden foods might be served. Cakes made with white flour were out, as were eggs. Chocolate in any form was strictly *verboten*.

Tommy did have some food allergies, but they were just a few of the many triggers for his asthma, and his mother's concern was out of proportion to his problems. As a result of her efforts, her family did learn good nutrition, but Tommy paid a heavy price. His brothers and sisters resented him, and his schoolmates called him "sissy." Unfortunately, by imposing her strong beliefs on everyone, Tommy's mother caused unnecessary dissension.

With counseling from her doctor, Tommy's mother became less strident in her approach. She provided Tommy with a special cupcake when he was invited to parties, and invited his friends to eat more often at his house. She even relented—although she did not change her views—and allowed her other children an occasional pizza and french fries.

Timothy

Timothy was typical of a great many young children with asthma. His family was very concerned about his disease, and hoped to protect him from any encounter that might trigger an attack. Every decision about his activities was made by someone else. He was quiet and withdrawn in school, and rarely volunteered to participate in any classroom group. Timmy's older sister attended the same school, and she would check on him several times a day. Timothy was afraid. He wasn't sure what or who the enemy might be, but he relied on his family to sort it out. Anytime he was without a family member he floundered. He did not understand his illness, and consequently was afraid of his own body. He had no confidence in his own instincts. Being near a child with a runny nose caused him to dissolve in tears. What would happen if he caught a cold? Would he have a severe attack? Unless given permission by his family to join in an activity, he was terrified to take a chance.

Once Timothy was encouraged to relax a little about his asthma, and once he understood what might trigger an attack, he became more self-confident. For the first time he really enjoyed school, games, and interaction with his schoolmates. Timmy's family had to learn how to step back and let Timothy become his own person.

Scott

Scott was caught between an overly concerned mother and a father who believed he was malingering. Scott's mother concentrated her full attention on Scott. However, she knew very little about his illness and worried most of the time about what "might happen." Scott's father was also deeply concerned about his son's illness; his method of coping with it was to deny it. He treated Scott's asthma like a football injury, and expected Scott to "walk it off." Scott felt guilty for causing his mother such obvious distress. He also felt inadequate to live up to his father's expectations. Too often his parents were locked in hot debate over the cause of Scott's asthma. All Scott wanted to do was breathe. However, the ugly fights caused stress, and Scott's asthma attacks increased in frequency and severity.

Education was the answer here. Once Scott and his family understood the true facts about asthma, and its causes and prevention, they were better equipped to control their own fears. Rather than wasting their energy arguing about Scott, they began to pull together to give Scott the positive support he needed.

None of the parents mentioned above wanted to intensify their children's problems, but all of them were so focused on listening to the wheeze that they forgot to listen to the child. Your child's illness isn't headline news. He deserves privacy. Share your concerns with each other or your doctor. Your child wants to be known for who he is, not for the illness he is struggling to overcome.

HOME:
THE LOCAL CLUBHOUSE

When our children were small, they often had to stay indoors during certain seasons of the year, and when the weather was bad. We turned our family room into a playroom, and encouraged their friends to come to our house to play. Along with the toys, puzzles, paints, and glue, we tried to provide a relaxed atmosphere so that the children would really enjoy playing there. We didn't interfere with their activities, and the rules of general cleanup were realistic—we didn't demand perfection.

As the children grew older, they still held events at our house. Pamela had many memorable parties. David's band rehearsed in the basement. Melissa's friends still assemble to watch MTV or movies. We've had the privilege of really knowing their friends, and still hear from many of them.

Slumber Parties

One of the more popular activities for children was exchanging overnight visits with their friends. When one of our children spent the night with a friend, or attended a slumber party, there were several procedures we followed. When they were young, I would call the friend's mother ahead of time, not to inventory her house for possible allergens but to let her know that she need not be overly concerned about our child's asthma. We would be at home, and the child had been instructed to call us immediately if any problems occurred. I wanted to reassure the mother that our child was just another guest, not a troubling responsibility. The children knew that if they had to be picked up during the night we would not be upset or annoyed. As a result, they never failed to call us if needed.

◊◊

> *I wasn't allowed to sleep over at some houses,*
> *because mothers feared I'd have an attack in*
> *their home. I hated that. It upset me more than*
> *when I was invited to a house and had to*
> *leave because I had an attack. No one ever*
> *tried to make me feel strange or odd, but I*
> *know that my asthma scared some. They*
> *didn't understand it and I couldn't explain it.*
>
> *—MELISSA*

It's No Big Deal

With friends and neighbors, we downplayed the children's asthma. It certainly wasn't the most important thing about them. We explained asthma wasn't contagious, it was totally reversible, and as the children grew older they would probably outgrow the symptoms. When we did run into a scout leader or soccer coach who was reluctant to have one of them in the group, we would tell the children it had nothing to do with them; the problem was a lack of information about asthma. We always managed to find an alternate troop or team, and the child had a better experience with a less anxious adult.

Butterflies flourish when wrapped in a cocoon. Children don't. If your child eats something he is allergic to at a friend's house or has an asthma attack while playing sports, attending a party, or vacationing, you know what medications to give him and where to go for additional medical help. The sky hasn't fallen, and he will be back to normal in a short time. Empathy for your child—putting yourself in his place—should dictate your reaction. He already has enough stress and embarrassment; don't add to it. A little flexibility and understanding is all it takes.

FAMILY: THE POWER OF LOVE

"If you were my wife, I would have left you!" This comment came from one of Melissa's doctors when he learned we had three asthmatic children. In one short sentence he reflected the attitude of many people faced with chronic illness. Blame someone else and distance yourself from responsibility. The disease becomes more important than the child, and the family collapses.

Positive Thinking

In our family, Gary's love, patience, and optimism set the tone from the beginning. His calm, positive approach to problems has made life more pleasant for all of us. I come from a family of inveterate worriers, and Gary helped me focus on solving problems rather than being overwhelmed by them. By learning all we could about asthma, and finding the best medical advice available, we have been able to view the children's disease in perspective. It became just one concern, not a major obstacle, in planning our family activities.

Our children were well aware of their asthma. They didn't need to be reminded of it over and over again. We have tried to control the disease, not the children. Constant questions concerning the children's health from well-meaning family and friends were discouraged by us. Pamela, David, and Melissa were normal, healthy children who occasionally had asthma. We have made the most of our wonderful asthma-free stretches.

Asthma was never used as an automatic reason to say "no" to proposed activities or adventures. The children knew how they were feeling, and we usually accepted their assessment of their capabilities. They didn't feel they were impaired, and I believe that many, many times their mental attitude played a large part in controlling their physical symptoms. Early in the game they took responsibility for taking their medication, and advising us when prescriptions at home or school needed refilling. Along with the normal fights and rivalries of siblings, a mutual caring for the well-being of each other has developed. They give each other support, not sympathy.

❁❁

My parents really taught us to handle asthma—to stay calm and mature—to tell people to call them. I always knew they would be there right away if I needed them.

—PAMELA

On Vacation

If the children's wheezing was somewhat under control, we would go ahead with plans for vacations and other extended activities. Realizing that changes in atmosphere, ocean breezes, and so forth might cause problems, we automatically got directions to the nearest local hospital when vacationing out of town. Then, if someone had an attack in the middle of the night, we would know exactly where to head for help. It was understood that if one of the children couldn't tolerate a new environment, we would immediately curtail the trip. Each of us knew that the child having difficulties didn't want to wheeze any more than we wanted to go home or to the hospital. We learned what *not* to say in those circumstances. No recriminations, no "if only's," and no undeserved feelings of guilt. Learning how to accept unavoidable disappointments with grace and understanding has been a valuable lesson that asthma has taught us all.

On the other hand, we didn't all stand around solicitously in the hospital room of the child suffering from asthma. Either Gary or I would stay with the one under attack. The others would head off to carry out vacation activities as planned.

The Holiday Seasons

Going to grandmother's for the holidays comes under the heading of a God-given right for a child. Unfortunately many holidays, from Halloween to the Fourth of July, coincide with seasonal weather changes. As so many asthmatics are adversely affected by these changes, joyous occasions can quickly turn to misery. Add the emotional baggage we all carry around during the expectant time before a big holiday, and you'll agree that a little planning and organization is worth it to prevent asthmatic episodes. Here is a list we always kept in mind:

1. Consult your journal and medical records for your child's asthmatic history for the time of year your trip is planned.

2. Contact your doctor and go over your child's asthmatic history with him. Ask him to suggest any medication adjustments or additions that might forestall wheezing.

3. Talk to the relatives or friends you are about to visit regarding environmental concerns (see chapter 7).

4. Limit your child's activities in the weeks before your trip to ensure proper rest.

5. Assemble all needed medications, medical equipment, and treatment letters in one box or small carrying case. Check expiration dates on medications. Carry new prescription orders with you if you think you may need refills during your trip. Be sure to pack this bag where it is easily accessible. If you are traveling by plane, *carry the bag with you*. Missing bags are bad enough without the accompaniment of an asthma attack.

6. If you are planning a long car trip, arrange to spend the night(s) with friends along the way or in a motel. It is important that your child arrive at your destination well rested, not overtired and cranky.

Twenty-four-hour car rides are pretty well guaranteed to ruin the rest of the trip.

7. Sit down with your child ahead of time, and calmly discuss some of the precautions he will have to take, and the behavior that will be expected of him. Cooperation in avoiding triggers will help eliminate nagging and anxiety.

8. Keep a turkey, or other appropriate holiday food, in the freezer or refrigerator. A last-minute cancellation need not totally spoil your celebration. Be prepared to take advantage of a fall-back position!

Sorry, We Can't Make It

Even with careful planning, we approached the holiday season holding our collective breath for many years. We prayed that the telltale dry cough and wheeze wouldn't develop. If it did, though, we knew that the child would be better off at home.

At such times, the acute disappointment of family and friends can make you feel like the Greek messenger who was killed for bringing bad news. Remember when you must make the dreaded cancellation call that the response may not be entirely sympathetic. You may be told your child doesn't eat right, doesn't sleep enough, is dressed too warmly, isn't dressed warmly enough, needs vitamins, takes too much medicine, has the wrong doctor, and so on. You may be given a dozen unrealistic suggestions on how to end the attack and salvage the trip.

You will need to be patient and understanding. Remember that what the speaker is after is a simple, immediate cure. Don't confuse this sincere caring with a personal attack. Worry and concern take many forms. It is not a good time to comment on the inappropriateness of the advice being offered.

Just listen! At the right moments you might slip in, "That's an interesting insight.... I'll look into that idea.... Thanks for mentioning that thought.... Noted!" Let the speaker feel helpful. It will make the disappointment easier to bear. Don't expect others to be knowledgeable as to all the intricacies of asthma. You know your child will be feeling better in a few hours or days. Hold that thought ... and do what you must.

WHEN HOME ISN'T QUITE ENOUGH

Asthmatic children need a great deal of resilience to deal with the complexities of their disease. Well one day and wheezing the next, they lead a roller-coaster existence. I have been amazed at my own children's ability to roll with the punches. Both Gary and I have tried to give them support and confidence, but I know sometimes all parents can do isn't enough. Let me tell you about two of the bravest children I have ever encountered in such a situation.

Cindy developed severe asthma as a toddler. Before she was four, she had experienced three tracheotomies. This procedure requires cutting a hole in the windpipe to facilitate breathing. The instability of Cindy's asthma caused numerous hospitalizations, some lasting as long as three to four weeks. The doctors were concerned that another tracheotomy would not be possible, due to the buildup of scar tissue within the small diameter of her windpipe.

Cindy required large doses of daily steroids, and while they were vital to her survival, we all knew the resulting side effects would take hold soon. The medications we take for granted today were not available when Cindy was small, and her medical team was constrained by what relief was available.

Dark curly hair, big brown eyes, and a lilting throaty laugh—that was Cindy. Even when the tracheotomies made speech impossible, she spoke to us with the twinkle in her eyes. Everyone loved her, and her cheerful, exuberant attitude infected the staff at the doctor's office and the hospital.

Cindy's difficulties would place a strain on any household. In Cindy's case the situation was complicated by a frequently bedridden mother and a traveling father. Too many times medicine was not given and minor attacks became emergencies.

As Cindy reached school age, her achievements in academics astounded everyone. Although she missed almost as many days of school as she attended, she was always near the top of her class and ready for more. Cindy had a smile on her face and a book in her hand at all times.

As school absences and hospitalizations increased, it became apparent to the doctors that intervention was necessary. After many consultations with Cindy's family and teachers, it was decided to send her to the Children's Asthma Research Institute and Hospital in Denver, Colorado. This facility has since merged with the National Jewish Center, and is now called the National Jewish Hospital for Immunology and Respiratory Medicine. The Institute offered a program for children with severe asthma to become residents of the hospital, where a treatment plan was worked out and each child was taught how to manage his own disease. While in residence they attended local Denver schools. The Institute paid most of the costs of transportation and residence, depending on the financial capabilities of the various families.

Cindy was in the fourth grade when she went to Denver. One of the specifications for treatment at the Institute at that time was called a "parentectomy," which meant no parental visits were permitted for at least eighteen months. In Cindy's case it was two years. This separation was intended to develop independence, and also to assure that the child was not pulled in opposite directions by two sets of authorities at the same time. Self-discipline in the severely diseased child is paramount, and Cindy learned self-discipline. (The Institute has since modified its approach, and allows parental involvement in a child's treatment, since research findings have made it clear it is the physiology of the child rather than the parents' psychological influence that causes asthma.)

Cindy's stories about her Denver experience were a mix of lamentation and delight. She had missed her family, but she was now able to understand and handle her own medications. She came to the office regularly for follow-ups and reported any change in her illness. She was no longer as dependent on steroids, and the new medications she took had no lasting side effects. She had enjoyed the "new" family she joined at the Institute. She reported some of the local Denver students resented the hospital "outsiders" joining their class. Names and sometimes spit balls were hurled in their direction. The hospital group bonded together as they plotted their revenge, and before long the two groups forgot their differences.

As Cindy grew older her attacks lessened, and cromolyn and the mist treatments taken with her portable compressor proved miracle workers in controlling her asthma. She continued to excel in school, took the Latin prize in her senior year of high school, and entered M.I.T. She is now working on her doctorate. And, oh yes, she occasionally wheezes.

Kevin could have listed his address as the local hospital. His asthma was so severe, and his attacks so frequent, that it seemed he only went home for visits! He was a slight child, almost constantly coughing, with sad, weary eyes.

Kevin's mother was a single parent. Her husband had difficulty holding on to his various jobs, and left the area. Kevin rarely saw his father, and was very protective of his mother. His mother usually worked at two or more jobs in order to provide for Kevin and herself. Visiting Kevin in the hospital was not easy for her. Her work load demanded many long hours, and she was dependent on public transportation. The separations caused by Kevin's many hospitalizations were emotionally devastating for both mother and child.

Because Kevin spent so much time in the hospital, he was far behind his peers in school. The county provided tutors who worked with him at the hospital, but he was usually too ill to keep up with school work.

When he did attend school he felt lost and frightened. His mother and doctors were all very concerned about his many unsupervised hours when he was at home. The doctors instructed their front desk employees to put through any call from Kevin immediately. When the situation showed no signs of improving, the doctors again contacted the Asthma Institute in Denver.

Kevin went to Denver when he was seven, and again when he was twelve. Kevin was not as outgoing as Cindy, and he had a difficult adjustment. Kevin's mother was finding the intricacies of Kevin's disease overwhelming. She had strong, deeply felt religious convictions and came to believe that Kevin's care should be in the hands of the Lord rather than medical advisors. Thus, his first trip to Denver was interrupted by his mother, who turned up unexpectedly and took him home. At about this time, cromolyn and other new medicines for asthma became available, and Kevin's mother was persuaded to include them in Kevin's treatment.

When Kevin was twelve he requested a return to Denver. This time he stayed the course, and learned to manage his own disease. His attitude changed as his health improved. Kevin began to feel comfortable and successful in his Denver school, and when he returned home he took a new interest in his local school. For the first time he was able to participate in intramural sports. He played soccer and football. By the time Kevin was sixteen he was six feet tall; fortunately his early dependence on steroids to control his asthma had not impeded his growth. Kevin's mother was so very proud of her son. She should have been. The source of much of the determination and strength he exhibited in overcoming his disease came from the spiritual guidance she provided.

As Kevin took more and more responsibility for his own treatment, he developed a strong interest in emergency medicine. He worked hard, and took all the courses necessary for certification in this field. I hope you will never need the rescue squad, but if you do, and a tall handsome young man is part of the team, his name might be Kevin.

A FAMILY THEME

I have heard a lot about "quality time" spent with children when it was convenient for parents and children to be together. As any parent of an asthmatic child knows, that kind of selective parenting is ludicrous. Our parenting is full-time, every day, throughout the nights, and all weekends, whether we're on the spot or have made extremely careful arrangements in our absence. The pressures of society to "live up to employment potential" do not take into consideration that all children are not healthy and rosy cheeked.

I will always be thankful for the years I spent with my children, and the close bond that we have for each other. Bonding takes place over many years, not in a "quality" moment.

As our children grew up, we pointed out life's possibilities, not its restrictions. I think this attitude helped give them confidence to try any activity that interested them. When asthma did limit their participation, we viewed it as a temporary setback. A gentle touch, an arm around the shoulder, a knowing, caring look, or a hug worked wonders for all of us when we were feeling down. During periods of physical inactivity, the children developed many intellectual, musical, and artistic talents they will continue to enjoy all their adult lives. Pamela has a deep love of literature. David has mastered the electric and acoustic guitar and the mandolin. Melissa's artistic abilities have earned her many awards, among them the countywide poster contest in parks and featured drawings in her high school's literary magazine. In sixth grade she won every weekly art contest in every category, to the point of such embarrassment that the teacher added new categories to spread the honors around.

We have encouraged each child's step forward on the way to controlling asthma. Two years ago Melissa was experiencing real difficulties with asthma—bad enough to force her to stay close to her home compressor. Today, thanks to treatment by Dr. Sly and her own positive approach toward handling the disease, her asthma is well under control.

About six months ago, Melissa phoned day and night in a successful effort to win tickets from a local radio station for a concert by Huey Lewis and the News. The seats she won were on the lawn of a huge outside pavilion in rural Maryland. *Lawn* was really a euphemism for an allotment of one individual per blade of grass. During the worst period of her asthma, she could never have attempted an evening on the lawn.

By the time we arrived, three quarters of the lawn was already filled with people, and our view was only of crowds in front of us. Nevertheless, we were singing and dancing and generally having a good time along with everyone else. Near the end of the concert, like Moses parting the Red Sea, the crowd moved apart and we could actually see the stage. Huey was performing his big hit, "The Power of Love." How beautifully appropriate, I thought. There's nothing like it.

10

❁ ❁ ❁

Adolescent Asthma

TEENAGE TROUBLES

Our children developed asthma in their very early childhood. Doctor visits, hospital stays, shots, allergy injections, and recurrent asthma attacks became a way of life. They accepted these difficulties as the norm, and assumed that everyone turned a little blue and wheezed on occasion.

As a child I don't think I even realized that my lungs functioned any differently than anyone else's. It wasn't as if I was cordoned off from people or activities because I was "asthmatic." Instead, I discovered through trial and error that certain stimuli set off reactions in my body that made it difficult to breathe, just as all children learn to respond to their environment.

—DAVID

However, I have met many children who have developed asthma later in childhood. Suddenly, they can no longer depend on their lungs. Running, biking, even walking can no longer be taken for granted. It is a very traumatic experience.

Hardest hit is the adolescent. Puberty, with all its glandular and hormonal changes, is a time of emotional stress for most young people. Add the manifestation of a chronic illness, and the result can be tragic. Just when independence and confidence are essential, they seem to lose both. Their friends and siblings are normal; they are strange. Often a child will try to deny his illness by refusing to take his medications or limit his activities. He becomes withdrawn and depressed. It is vital that this reaction be turned around. While we're talking here about the teenager just getting asthma, it's obvious that much of this information can apply as well to a child with a history of asthma who is now taking on the turmoil of adolescence.

Looking back, I realize the illness really ran my life. It prevented me from being as spontaneous as I wanted to be. I couldn't run the 600 or the 50-yard dash during physical fitness testing. Friends used to tell me I was lucky. I never felt lucky. I felt awkward and left out.

—MELISSA

Preparing to Fight Back

If your newly asthmatic child is in junior high or high school, speak with his school counselor. The counselor can advise his teachers so they will be aware of his health and emotional concerns. Since many absences may result from your child's asthma, support from his teachers is a necessity. Falling behind in school can cause feelings of depression and rejection to deepen.

The young person must become well educated about his particular triggers, and learn how to avoid developing attacks. The best place to start this education is at your doctor's office. You may have noticed that sometime after your child's seventh birthday the level of your wisdom and common sense dropped in inverse proportion to his age! Obviously whatever advice you have to give is open to question. On the other hand, he may listen to a health professional.

Your child will benefit from establishing a close relationship with his doctor and staff. Arrange an appointment for this purpose as soon as possible. At this appointment your doctor might provide:

1. A thorough explanation of asthma: its causes and effects—an overview of the basic nature of the disease.

2. Statistics on the prevalence of the disease in the population, emphasizing how common asthma is in the child's age group. The child should be assured that asthma is a completely reversible disease. He needs to understand that no long-lasting damage is

being done to his lungs, and with proper treatment and his wholehearted cooperation he can expect a full and active life.

3. An explanation of the child's own role in reaching control, letting him know that his help in managing his asthma is the most important element in his treatment plan.

4. A detailed description of the medications he will be taking: what effect each medication will have on his asthma, what side effects may be expected, exact dosage to be taken, how often the medication should be taken. He should get the message that the combination of these medications constitutes a prescribed treatment plan that will bring about desired results in relieving asthmatic symptoms if followed carefully.

5. Encouragement for the child to ask any and all questions he may have relative to his asthma.

It is important that neither parent act as a buffer between doctor and child at this meeting, or indeed at future appointments. The child and his doctor should be allowed to deal with each other directly. If the child is self-assured, parents can stay out of the first session entirely. The child needs to feel comfortable and compatible with his doctor, much like the relationship between a coach and team member. You'll get the scoop on the essentials that were discussed when you talk with them after the appointment.

Friendly Persuasion

Nothing is more important to the teenager than the respect and acceptance of his peers. Dr. Sly and his medical staff at Children's Hospital understand this need. Periodic rap sessions are held with these teenaged asthma patients. At these sessions, anxieties, fears, and anger are voiced. As each child reveals his feelings, he is helping other children understand they are not isolated by their disease, and a network of support is developed. They help each other react to the pressures of friends and parents, often with humor.

They learn from this exposure to other asthmatics that most actually do improve. They also are able to discuss their fears with health professionals in a relaxed atmosphere. Questions they might be too self-conscious to ask in a more formal setting are easier to broach.

If your doctor does not already have classes and training sessions for parents and children, suggest that such support groups be formed. The older children can help develop guidelines for younger asthmatics that can help them approach their teenage years more successfully. It is a secondary benefit of a successful support group, but an important one.

Depending on the severity of your child's asthma, and his reaction to the disruption it causes, professional counseling may be called for. A few sessions with a trained therapist may save your child much heartache. In fact, the whole family may benefit from a session where they are involved. Gaining a good perspective on how to handle the physical and psychological problems of being asthmatic is the key to successful treatment.

It is important to keep in mind that while puberty often brings marked improvement in asthmatic symptoms, it can also cause some children's asthma to become unstable. Don't be discouraged if this happens. Often the medications must be adjusted or supplemented during these years. Stay in close contact with your doctor, and be sure your child understands the dynamics of the normal body changes at this time. The problems, properly handled, will most likely be temporary.

> *Having asthma has made me a stronger, more caring and accepting person. I am able to deal with disappointments more readily and I have learned from my mistakes. I think having asthma has made me a better person. It has helped make me who I am today. Since I was a little girl, I have had to make others feel at ease with my illness. I think this is why I get along well with many different kinds of people. I have had to emphasize my strengths to compensate for the limitations of my illness. This has given me a great deal of confidence in myself and my abilities.*
>
> *—MELISSA*

THE QUESTION GAME

Q: *"Hey, man, why you taking all that medicine? What's that stuff in the inhaler? Are you a druggie?"*
A: *"Listen, dude, this stuff's called breathing. Blue's not my best color!"*

Q: *"Did you take your medicine today?"*
A: *"Okay, Mom, let's make a great compromise. You can ask me just once a week if I've taken my medication, and I'll keep taking it every day. Deal?"*

Q: *"Is asthma psychosomatic?"*
A: *"No, but I really wish it was. If it was all in my mind I could think it away!"*

Q: *"Will you outgrow your asthma?"*
A: *"I'm definitely planning on it!"*

Q: *"Are you going to die?"*
A: *"For sure. Probably at ninety, listening to music."*

If these responses seem glib, that's not the intention. Usually the questioner is not looking for a detailed answer, just reassurance for his own anxiety. Frequently, a humorous, lighthearted reply lets him know the young person is on top of the problem and not unduly concerned. At rap sessions or asthma classes, the youngsters might be encouraged to play the "Question Game." It helps them become more comfortable talking about their illness, and they learn not to take themselves or their disease too seriously.

Of course, your child can only project this attitude if he feels confident of his ability to cope with his asthma. Confidence only comes through education. Your child must fully understand the causes (triggers) of his asthma, the limitations it imposes, and what medications he is using to control it.

Let's be honest. The worst of asthma can be very bad. Here, Melissa looks back on an attack that threatened her life when she was seventeen. It is important to know some of the feelings that a teenager with severe asthma experiences.

Asthma: A Slow Take

The alarm clock rings,
    But I am already awake.
A gauze-like sunlight streams through my window,
    Shining on my peach prom dress—
    Still glowing from the weekend.
The room looks olive through the transparent green mask I wear.
The familiar rumble of my breathing machine pumps the white mist of medicine through the mask,
    Making the room foggy.
My lungs make a screaming noise from within,
    They are crying.
They are asking,
    "Why did you go to that dance, instead of to the doctor like your parents said?"
My mother comes into the room,
    She can hear my lungs—
    But she can't understand what they are saying.
Looking at my sunken, exhausted body she doesn't say,

"I told you so."—
She probably doesn't even think it.

Instead she whispers, "They're on their way."
The room starts to spin—
I wonder if I will die.

Secretly, I hope death will end my suffocation.
Why did I let myself get so sick?

The paramedics arrive,
And they look like two big faces staring at
me.

It seems as if I'm filming a movie,
And they are looking right into my camera.

"Do you feel faint?"
One of them asks.

I shake my head,
Right before I black out.

—MELISSA B. STEVENS

11

Sports and Exercise

"WINNING" AT SPORTS FOR THE ASTHMATIC

The emphasis on physical fitness so prevalent in the country today is not a new concept in America. Theodore Roosevelt, our twenty-sixth president, believed that physical fitness and the "strenuous life" were important national goals. He popularized physical activity by his own example. He hiked, camped, boxed, rowed, played tennis, swam, rode horseback, climbed mountains—with vigor.

Teddy was an asthmatic. He developed severe asthma in early childhood, and wheezed his way into adolescence. As a teenager he was determined to control his disease through body-building exercises. He was successful because he had the determination and desire to participate in daily exercise and sports.

Today, new medications, especially cromolyn and beta-agonist inhalers, make athletic activities much easier for asthmatics. The essential ingredient, though, is still the child's desire to participate. Children rarely choose to be physically active because of potential benefits to their lungs and general muscle tone. They participate because they want to play. Parents should let their children choose their favorite activities, and then support that participation.

Cold-weather sports are not out of the question for asthmatics, though chilly, dry weather is not the climate of choice. They can warm the air they're breathing by wrapping a scarf around the face. Exercises illustrated later in this chapter that teach them to breathe from the diaphragm, rather than sucking air in through the mouth, also help in the cold weather.

Given time, active sports can make a difference. In studies by Dr. François Haas of New York University Hospital, sedentary people with asthma lost 30 percent of their lung capacity after exercise. Following three months of regular workouts, their lung capacity dropped only 10 percent after exercise.

Children with exercise-induced asthma often have difficulties eight to ten minutes into any kind of physical activity. Inhalation of a beta-agonist such as albuterol not only helps prevent exercise-induced asthma for four to six hours but also improves airway size to lessen the adverse effect of a small amount of obstruction induced by exercise. Your child should take cromolyn one-half hour before physical exertion to gain this advantage. Children who experience sporadic wheezing—not every time they exercise—are often helped by inhalers. Theophylline, taken before exercise, works for others. Sometimes a combination of these medications is the answer.

The warm-up period before the main event is important for any athlete, but especially so for the asthmatic child. Moving into strenuous exercise gradually can minimize the asthma that occurs after more sustained activity.

Pulmonary function tests are an extremely useful tool in determining which medications are most effective for your child. The tests assess the child's lung capacity, and the degree of airway restriction during exercise. When taking such a test, the child runs in place, or around the doctor's office, simulating strenuous activity. The effect on the lungs and airways is measured before and after running, and before and after medication is taken. This information helps the doctor in determining the best medications to control or prevent exercise-induced asthma.

When your child is able to participate more fully in sports and exercise, the emotional benefits match the physical ones. David, who earned the Presidential Physical Fitness Award and set five field-day track records in sixth grade, went on to enjoy many sports in high school and college. He still lifts weights regularly. Pamela, who wheezed so badly as a little girl, played soccer throughout high school. Her inhaler was always part of her equipment. Sometimes she played the whole game, if she was wheezy she played at short intervals. But she always played.

Melissa took part in swimming, which is an ideal

sport for asthmatics, since it increases lung capacity at the same time it exercises almost all of the important body muscles. Swimming meets are judged not just on speed but on the accuracy of the stroke. During practice, children swim many laps of the backstroke, free style, breast stroke, and butterfly. The weekly meetings and ribbon presentations are wonderful fun for the whole family, but the real prize is won at the daily practices. Actually, the same is true of all sports activities.

WHAT ABOUT SUMMER CAMPS?

In the spring of Melissa's seventh-grade year, plans for the coming summer were the hot topic of conversation among Melissa and her friends. As they discussed possibilities (too young to drive, too young to work, and too old, they felt, to hang around the neighborhood pool) the option of two weeks of summer camp was high on their list. Melissa was caught up in the enthusiasm, even though her asthma was not fully under control. She carried on a strong campaign to convince her parents and her doctors that she could handle it. Eventually she wore us down, and I contacted the camp her friends were considering to discuss her health needs. Although they didn't have specially trained personnel for individual diseases, they assured me there was a daytime doctor and a nighttime nurse available. With some apprehension I sent in her deposit.

As luck and the "asthma gods" would have it, Melissa's asthma became more and more unstable as spring turned into summer. Instead of two weeks at summer camp she found herself in the pediatric intensive care unit of our local hospital on a respirator. The folks at the camp were very understanding, and sent back our deposit. However, for Melissa the disappointment of not being able to go to camp lasted a long time. She wanted so much to be able to make normal commitments like all her friends—not to have to weigh all the pros and cons and deal with "are they equipped to handle?" considerations.

I really believe we let Melissa down badly in our willingness to agree. We wanted the norm for her too, but her reality dictated otherwise. A study published in the *Journal of the American Medical Association* in May 1990 pointed out that asthma deaths are 13 percent higher in summer than during the rest of the year. One assumption is that children are more likely to be on their own in these months, and they may not get attention fast enough, which could be a problem at a camp not equipped to manage asthma.

Today I think we could give a better response to Melissa's request, thanks to the availability of more than eighty camps throughout the country designed for asthmatic children. A little careful research on your part can lead to a wonderful summer experience for your child. These camps not only provide exercise and outdoor fun but they schedule asthma self-help classes where children learn from experts and each other how to manage their disease.

Dr. Mark Holbreich and Dr. Stephen C. Weisberg have written a definitive article on this subject, a must-read for parents of any camp-bound child with more than mild asthma: "Asthma Camp: Whom to Send, What to Look For," *The Journal of Respiratory Diseases*, April 1990. You can find this magazine in any local library or in your doctor's office.

The benefits of going to camp, both physical and psychological, are analyzed, along with potential drawbacks. Valuable check lists and what to look for and ask about are fully discussed. Camp can help give our asthmatic children some of the independence they are striving for, and this article supplies the guidance parents need in selecting the right environment. At the end of this highly informative article is a list of asthma camps.

RELAAAX!

With regard to any kind of exercise, the main obstacle confronting the asthmatic child is not the wheezing episode that strenuous activity might cause. It is the restrictions imposed by concerned and fearful parents. Frequently those limitations are placed on the child because of anticipated problems rather than real ones. Give your children the opportunity to take part in all the activities of childhood. Expend your energy in making the needed adjustments and arrangements to make these activities possible rather than in unnecessary worrying. Overly concerned parents teach their child to be afraid of his own body, and the child grows up without the confidence to face new challenges.

The child himself can also benefit from exercise to

lessen physical and emotional tension. Relaxation exercises not only help relax constricted muscles but they allow the child to have control over his body. This control reduces much of the fear an asthmatic experiences during an acute attack, and teaches him the positive results of true self-discipline.

The choice of relaxation exercises depends on the age and interests of the child. They vary from simple to complex. Information should be available at your doctor's office. Your physician can start your child off with basic breathing exercises. A printed instruction sheet with pictures of each exercise will be a helpful reference, but be sure your doctor or a member of their staff demonstrates the procedure for your child first, and then observes the child practicing the exercise. Your doctor can also refer you to a specialist in this field who can offer more sophisticated training in such methods as meditation, biofeedback, yoga, hypnosis, guided imagery, or physical therapy.

During the television coverage of the 1984 Olympics there were several interviews with sports psychologists. Of particular interest was the method used to help an injured athlete stay in shape. The athlete was taught how to concentrate on his body and was taken mentally through his regular practice exercises, thus making his muscles respond as if he were actually doing the workout.

Many relaxation techniques use this principle in reverse. The child is taught how to concentrate on a pleasant experience or activity. During periods of stress, such as an asthma attack, the imagery training allows the child to concentrate on a calm, relaxing event, and the constricted muscles relax. This method, very effective for many children, can be taught with relatively few lessons.

Once your child has chosen his favorite sport(s), and found ways to overcome the barriers that asthma places in the way of taking part in the activity, he will be much more certain that he, rather than his asthma, is going to be in charge of his body.

> I had a normal life—soccer, aerobics, everything. Asthma just gets in the way at times. If you give in to it . . . then you give in to it . . . and you just can't do that.
>
> —PAMELA

Breathing Treatments

Another form of exercise for the asthmatic child is the use of techniques specifically designed to improve breathing. These range from postural drainage processes that remove mucus from the air passages of the lungs to breathing exercises that make a child more conscious of the way his lungs, along with his chest and stomach muscles, can best work together to facilitate better breathing. The following illustrations can give you and your child a start. Other books on the list in the appendix go into more detail.

WHAT IS POSTURAL DRAINAGE?

Postural drainage is a technique that uses positioning to help remove mucus from the air passages of the lungs. Percussion (clapping) over specific areas of the chest with a cupped hand will help dislodge the mucus from the small air passages, which will then allow the child to cough up the mucus more easily.

These two procedures will help the child to clear his lungs of mucus and should be used when you find that your child is coughing more frequently or that the amount of mucus has increased. The figures represented below will help properly position your child.

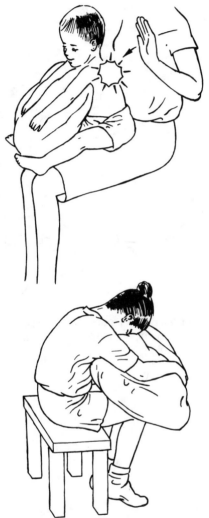

Position: Your child is sitting, leaning forward over pillows. Clap on both sides of the upper back.

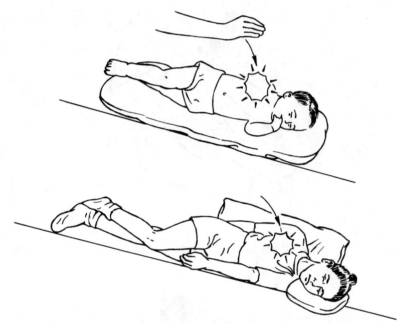

Position: Your child lies on his left side. Place a pillow behind him from the shoulders to the hips and have him roll slightly back on it. Clap over the right nipple.

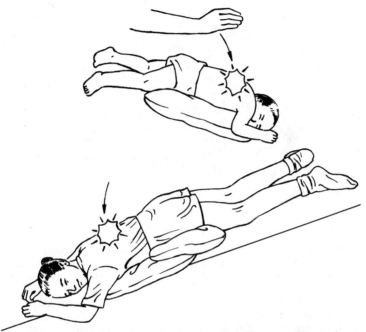

Position: Have your child lie on his right side. Place a pillow in front and have him roll slightly forward onto it. Clap at the lower ribs and middle back. Repeat above, except this time your child should lie on his left side.

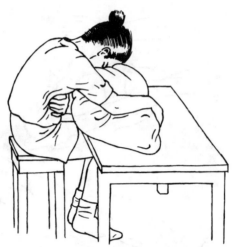

If your child has difficulty breathing, have him sit comfortably forward on a chair beside a table on which he can rest his arms and relax his upper chest. Have him hold his stomach with one hand. As he breathes in through his nose, he should feel his stomach push out against his hand. As he breathes out through his mouth, his stomach should sink in.

This exercise should be done at the child's own rate, and once he gains control of this pattern of breathing, then you should encourage him to slow down his rate.

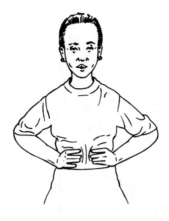

EXERCISES TO HELP YOUR CHILD
IMPROVE HIS BREATHING

Basic Starting Exercise

1. Have your child sit erect on the edge of his bed or chair and place his hands over his lower ribs and upper abdomen. He should keep his shoulders down, elbows straight out, fingers rigid.
2. Have him exhale while he applies firm pressure against his ribs and abdomen with his hands. He should exhale through pursed lips . . . lips held as though he is about to whistle.
3. He should inhale after releasing pressure of hands slightly, but still apply effort against his chest and abdomen. Ask him to cough gently to bring up phlegm. Then repeat ten times or as your doctor directs.

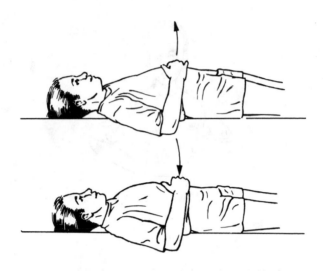

Exercise 2

1. Have your child lie flat on the floor, resting his left hand across his chest, his right hand on his abdomen.
2. Have him inhale deeply through his nose, letting his abdomen rise.
3. Have him breathe out through pursed lips, pressing his abdomen firmly up toward his chest. He should try to move his chest as little as possible and let his abdomen move up and down as he inhales and exhales. Have him repeat this exercise six to eight times. Once he has developed this breathing technique he should try to breathe in this way even while walking.

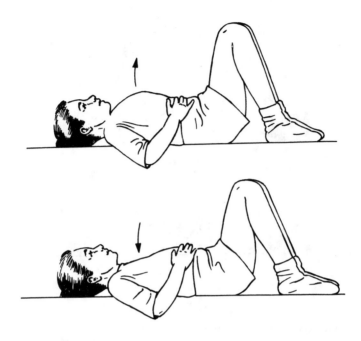

Exercise 3

1. Have your child lie flat on the floor resting his left hand across his chest, his right hand on his abdomen.
2. Have him bend his knees as shown in the picture, keeping his knees close together and his feet flat on the floor.
3. He should inhale through his nose, letting his abdomen rise against his right hand.
4. He should exhale through pursed lips (as though he was whistling), pressing in and up on his abdomen. Have him repeat six to eight times or as your doctor directs.

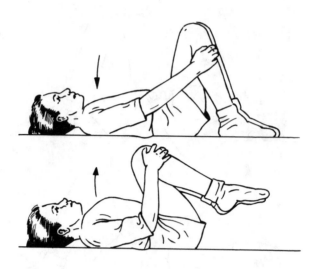

Exercise 4

1. Have your child lie flat on the floor.
2. Have him bend his knees and lock his arms around his legs.
3. He should inhale through his nose, letting his abdomen rise.
4. He should then lift his feet from the floor and exhale through pursed lips, pulling his knees toward his chest as far as possible. Have your child repeat this exercise six to eight times or as your doctor directs.

Adapted with the kind permission of the Johns Hopkins Children's Center.

CHAPTER

12

✿ ✿ ✿

Financing This Disease

To "all you can count on is death and taxes," parents of asthmatics can add medical bills. We don't have to check the government list of leading economic indicators to know the cost of medical services has skyrocketed in recent years. Most of us feel that we have personally endowed our doctors' offices and put their children through college! Since the need for medical care and prescription drugs is ongoing, the financial strain on the family budget is awesome. The stress of outstanding medical bills, added to continuing health problems, can be overwhelming. Where do you turn for help?

A DOLLAR HERE, A DOLLAR THERE

No one is more aware of the high cost of chronic illness than your doctor. Don't hesitate to discuss payment plans with your physician. Agree on a mutually acceptable minimum monthly payment arrangement. Be sure you send that amount each month, and larger payments when possible. It will relieve your anxiety over doctor bills, while showing your good faith in meeting your financial obligations. As your child's health improves, so will your ability to reduce outstanding medical debts.

If your child is taking daily medication on a continuing basis, check with your pharmacist on the most economical quantity to order. Share this information with your doctor, and ask them to write future prescriptions for this amount. When your child is starting a new medication, ask to be started off with samples to be sure your child will tolerate the new drug before you fill a prescription. Request the use of generic drugs when appropriate; they are less expensive than brand-name drugs. (*Note:* Different brands of slow-release theophylline preparations have vastly different effects, so they should never be used interchangably or interdependently.)

Insurance Choices

Medical insurance coverage is often dictated by what plan your employer carries. However, if you are in a position to choose options, study the specific services offered very carefully before selecting a carrier or a plan for your family. Don't choose your coverage based on overall cost alone. Your child may be hospitalized frequently. What is the deductible charge for each admission before coverage begins? Are asthma attacks considered a medical emergency? Are allergy workups and shots covered? Is home medical equipment covered? What is the reimbursement for prescription drugs? How large is the yearly individual deduction for each family member before medical coverage begins? Are preexisting medical problems covered by a new carrier? Can you select your own doctors?

If you are considering HMO (Health Maintenance Organization) coverage, keep in mind that most HMOs require you to use doctors employed by their group. Visit the facility and interview the supervising physician. Ask how a chronic illness is handled, and be sure your child won't be seeing a different doctor every time he wheezes. Find out if an allergy/asthma specialist is on staff, and if he will be seeing your child regularly. Is a wheezing child seen immediately without an appointment? Always ask about their referral policy: Will they cover charges for services not provided on the premises? Will your child be referred to a specialist if needed? Can you select the specialist? Be sure the hospital where the HMO group has privileges is easily accessible to you in emergency situations. Arrange an appointment with the physician who will be treating your child's asthma. Go over your child's asthmatic history with this doctor, and be sure that his expectation for control, choice of treatment plans, and general outlook are compatible with yours.

If you are considering a PPO (Preferred Provider Organization), ask for a list of affiliate physicians in your area. With this plan you can select your own doctors from the list of those affiliated with the plan. Carefully study the benefits offered, and ask any questions you might have about the coverage with one of the doctors on the list. Many HMOs and PPOs offer standard and high-option medical plans. Find out what major medical expenses the higher option covers, and how much more are the monthly charges. It may provide much better coverage with only a slight increase in cost.

When considering a change from one insurance plan to another, be sure the new carrier will cover costs for preexisting medical problems. My advice is to get this commitment in writing from the insurance company, or its agent, before you make any changes. Otherwise you could end up with no coverage at all for your asthmatic child.

The Bottom Line

Melissa was always in the hospital. The financial constraints were terrible. I could see it was hard on my parents. I don't know how they stood it.

—PAMELA

The many medical bills that accompany chronic illness make discussions about disposable income unnecessary. From personal experience, I know how quickly those medical bills dispose of all income. We learned that patio building, carpet and furniture shopping, new cars, and designer wardrobes weren't for us. When we did take vacations, they were simple excursions to the nearest beach. However, we knew we had no choice and we agreed on what our priorities were. A healthy child came first; that was always the bottom line. The pressures and tensions caused by ever-mounting medical expenses can be terrible, but keep your eyes on the end result.

In the last few years there have been many proposals for profound changes in the healthcare delivery system for the nation. Medical and insurance costs have become so high that a thorough look at the system is appropriate. More emphasis on preventive medicine is certainly necessary. However, we must be careful that cost-cutting proposals don't result in a lowering in the quality of care our children receive. Insurance costs, both to doctors and patients, are becoming prohibitive, and action is needed. The bottom line, though, must represent the best care available, not just the lowest cost.

My father once told me the best investment I would ever make was in my children's health. Although he never envisioned how large this investment was to be, I have come to respect and appreciate his philosophy. Everything else is secondary. Fortunately, asthma is a treatable disease, and with the proper medical care the prognosis is excellent. The sooner you provide your child with the best medical support available, the shorter his asthmatic ordeal will be.

13

❁ ❁ ❁

Strength in Numbers: Getting Together to Fight Asthma

You are not alone. It may seem so when your child is gasping for air at 3 A.M., but the fact is there are hundreds of thousands of parents like you, looking for that delicate mixture of medication and positive attitude that will keep a child well. They like to get together to share experiences, advice, doctors' names, and all the small triumphs and tragedies that accompany the growing-up years, with or without asthma.

We are fortunate that the National Heart, Lung and Blood Institute (NHLBI) at the National Institutes of Health (NIH) has focused direct attention on the problems surrounding asthma. As they have with other health issues like smoking, high blood pressure, and cholesterol, they have mounted a National Asthma Education Program. The program has three goals:

1. To raise awareness of patients, health professionals, and the public that asthma is a serious chronic disease.
2. To ensure the recognition of the symptoms of asthma by patients, families, and the public and the appropriate diagnosis by health professionals.
3. To ensure effective control of asthma by encouraging a partnership among patients, physicians, and other health professionals through modern treatment and education programs.

The program operates on the premise, proven in several random controlled studies, that patient education programs effectively reduce the number of asthma attacks, emergency room visits, and hospitalizations, particularly in previously hospitalized children. Days lost from school decrease and school grades improve. The studies also show that education programs significantly reduce healthcare costs in high-risk populations.

Several private, public, and voluntary health organizations as well as federal agencies, including the National Institute of Allergy and Infectious Diseases have come together to form the National Asthma Education Program Coordinating Committee. This committee is coordinated by the NHLBI.

A total of twenty-seven national associations and federal agencies are working on coordinated educational approaches. Some are for medical professionals; some are for patients and their families; some are for schools. All of the organizations mentioned in this chapter are benefiting from both the attitude and the money involved in this program.

The program has been in place a relatively short time, but various educational resources are being developed. Write to Robinson Fulwood, Coordinator, National Asthma Education Program, Building 31, Room 4A18, Bethesda, MD 20892.

When you're looking for the kind of activity or support that only a mutual-interest group can offer, you might try some of the following associations.

ASTHMA & ALLERGY
FOUNDATION OF AMERICA

This organization (1717 Massachusetts Ave., N.W., Suite 305, Washington, DC 20036) has a growing number of programs aimed at asthmatics and their families. Their ambitious mission is to "help find the cure for, and ultimately eradicate, asthma and other allergic diseases." In the meantime, they want to "serve the estimated 35 million victims of asthma and other allergic diseases through support of education, research, and service programs."

The Asthma & Allergy Foundation supports the formation of local support groups. You may find one already in operation in your area. If not, you can order a "Support Group Resource Kit," a package of print and audiotape materials that suggest everything from icebreakers for the first meeting to how to obtain free radio and cable advertising.

For schools, the Foundation offers a training manual called "Asthma in the School." It concentrates on the benefits of peak flow monitoring, and gives school nurses instructions on the use of the peak flowmeter. Worth their weight in gold are sample school forms and sample letters between school, parent, and doctor that will be needed when developing effective treatment for students with asthma.

Perhaps the most exciting program sponsored by the Asthma & Allergy Foundation is ACT (Asthma Care Training). This program is for parents and their six- to twelve-year-old children. It increases their knowledge of symptoms, causes, and treatments for asthma; explores their feelings about the disease; and gives them better control over ways to prevent asthmatic episodes.

At a series of weekly sessions, children and parents meet separately for a training period, then unite for the remaining time to share their experiences. The training team includes four individuals: a program coordinator, a parents' group teacher, a children's group teacher, and a physician or pharmacist—who are in turn trained by regional experts on the staff.

ACT uses lots of drawings, charts with stickers, and games to keep kids' interests from flagging. This active program assures that both children and parents learn the ABCs of handling asthma, and emphasizes the benefits of children taking over as much of their own care as possible.

In addition to these programs, the Foundation offers brochures, books, and manuals on everything from "Teaching Myself About Asthma" to "Quackery and Questionable Treatment in Asthma and Allergy Medicine." Write them for a listing.

AMERICAN LUNG ASSOCIATION

The American Lung Association (ALA) adopted a special three-year nationwide focus on asthma in 1990. This organization also addresses other lung health issues such as smoking, air pollution, emphysema, and lung cancer. They have concluded that the increases in sickness and death caused by asthma, together with advances in the ability to treat it, make it particularly timely to educate people who may not have been diagnosed as yet, or are not getting complete treatment.

ALA has a chapter in every state, plus some local affiliates in more populous regions. Check your phone book for the one nearest you, or contact the national organization at: 1740 Broadway, New York, NY 10019-7374 (212-315-8700).

Each state and local group determines what programs to offer, but each is increasing their emphasis on asthma in some way. This might include support groups, summer camp programs, training for school personnel and health care professionals, outreach to minority communities, publications, and workshops for patients and families.

Among the materials offered nationwide by ALA is a kit called "Superstuff," which provides the younger child with puzzles, stories, riddles, and games designed to help him understand his disease and to encourage his self-confidence in dealing with attacks. An exciting new ALA initiative is "Open Airways for Schools." This is a special ALA adaptation of a successful program for children with asthma aged eight to eleven, developed by Columbia University's College of Physicians and Surgeons. It consists of six group sessions held during the school day. The program is led by a trained instructor who could be a classroom teacher, school nurse, health educator, or Lung Association volunteer. The ALA's goal is to ensure that quality asthma health education is available in the school setting for every child with asthma. "Open Airways for Schools" was piloted in four states in 1990, with nationwide availability planned for late 1991.

MOTHERS OF ASTHMATICS, INC.

Founded by Nancy Sander, a dynamic young mother of an asthmatic, she has become well known as a leader in the fight against asthma. Mothers of Asthmatics, Inc. defines itself as a "support system in a newsletter." It does not organize group activities, but acts as a clearinghouse, pulling together information from a number of sources to report in its monthly newsletter, "M. A. Report." You can receive this eight-page (no advertising) publication for $25 per year.

Mothers of Asthmatics also offers discounts on peak flowmeters. They sell the "Asthma Organizer," a home diary system especially helpful to families whose children have been diagnosed but do not yet have their asthma under control. Their doctors want to know every detail possible about day-to-day symptoms and treatment. The Asthma Organizer helps.

M. A., Inc. offers children's books—*So You Have Asthma, Too* and *I'm a Meter Reader*—for children four to ten years old. A video is available to accompany *So You Have Asthma, Too*.

Write to: Mothers of Asthmatics, Inc., 10875 Main Street, Suite 210, Fairfax, VA 22030 for more information, or call: 703-385-4403, or 1-800-878-4403.

Conferences on Asthma

Watch for conferences you can attend that tell you more about asthma and give you a chance to talk with others about problems and solutions in fighting it. In 1990, the American College of Allergy & Immunology presented a series of conferences, "Conquer Your Asthma . . . Control Your Life." For a registration fee of only $30, the conferences presented the latest proven and preferred asthma management techniques, with emphasis on practical applications for home, work, and school. Allergists and other health-care professionals discussed and answered questions on all aspects of asthma. While no specific sessions were scheduled at the time this book went to press, signs point to the availability of more conferences like these in the future.

Just for Fun

An annual Asthma Ski Day is held each spring in Beaver Creek, Colorado, for asthmatics from seven to seventeen years old and their families (adult members of families are welcome). Activities range from lessons for beginners to races for the swift. Medical supervisors teach asthmatics how to participate in cold-weather activities with as little interference from their disease as possible.

You've probably already been surprised that just about everyone who hears your child has asthma can tell you of a member in their own family who has—or once had—asthma. The grassroots movement is sweeping America, encouraging people to take control of their lives and to work together to improve them. Why should asthmatics be any different? Groups can lobby, advise, and obtain expert help in ways you can't do alone—not to mention the lifelong friendships they offer. Think about joining one.

14

✿ ✿ ✿

What Does
The Future Hold?

There have been so many exciting developments in the control of asthma during the three decades my children have faced it. At the same time, it has become a more general, and sometimes more serious, disease. What can we look for in the next ten years or so in the fight against asthma?

When I put this question to Melissa's Dr. Sly, a nationally known expert on childhood asthma, his response wasn't exactly what I expected. He told me that the Waorani Indians inhabit a 620-square-mile protectorate in a rain forest at the headwaters of the Amazon River in eastern Ecuador. They live in temporary shelters made of palm leaves and wood, scattered through the jungle near gardens where they grow bananas and a few other crops. Although they lack comfortable beds and shiny cars, they also miss the associated house dust mites and air pollutants. And they have no asthma!

Physicians who studied the Waorani a few years ago found only two who had mild allergic rhinitis, and those two happened to be the only inhabitants who had traveled extensively to the Ecuadorian capital of Quito and to the United States and Europe. It seems that the environment, rather than a genetic predisposition, has protected the Waorani.

The mystery seemed to deepen as Dr. Sly talked on. He said that the two Waorani who exhibited allergies had eaten beef for the first time in their travels, while monkey had been their chief previous source of meat. He mentioned that asthma has been very infrequent in societies where fish has been a major source of protein, and that within a few weeks a daily dietary supplement of fish oil can have a potentially beneficial effect on the type of chemicals released by allergic reactions (although he warns that studies are still needed to see whether large amounts of fish oil might have other, less desirable effects on health). Intriguing as these observations are, short-term trials of dietary supplementation with fish oil in asthmatic patients have failed to cause any negligible lessening of symptoms.

What Dr. Sly was getting at, I found, was a suggestion that changes in lifestyle may become more and more important in controlling asthma. Ever the good scientist, Dr. Sly is not about to leap to conclusions about this or that possible environmental cause of asthma. But he did say changes that have occurred in the same population over time help to divide possible environmental effects from genetic influences. Giving another example, he said in 1962 asthma was unknown in certain villages in Papua, New Guinea, but within ten years more than 7 percent of the adults in the same villages had asthma. What happened? During this same decade these people had begun to use blankets. Their blankets were found to be heavily infested with the same kinds of mites that contribute the most important allergens to house dust. Almost all the people with asthma were extremely allergic to these mites—a source of allergens virtually ubiquitous in Western civilization. Exposure to this source of potent allergens may have caused the asthma.

As I indicated in chapter 7 on the environment, relatively modest changes in the bedroom can greatly reduce exposure to mites. Acarosan can kill mites that infest carpeting, and Allergy Control Solution can inactivate mite allergens. An agent sold in Europe called *primiphos methyl* also kills mites in carpets and upholstered furniture.

The new laws and social norms related to the surgeon general's goal of a smoke-free society may also decrease the prevalence as well as the severity of childhood asthma, since passive exposure to smoking worsens the disease.

In the area of drugs, Dr. Sly says that longer-acting, more effective drugs will become available within the next decade. Some will act in different ways from those now in use. Ipratropium bromide, long available in Canada and Europe and available in the United States in metered dose inhalers, improves lung function in some asthmatics through a mechanism different from that of other drugs aimed at relieving airway obstruction.

As has been true in recent years, additional drugs coming on the market will allow drug combinations that will make control of asthma with drugs more simple. Dr. Sly says the introduction of antihistamines with fewer side effects may permit use of doses large enough to help control asthma, as well.

Treatment with allergy injections will soon be safer, more effective, and more convenient. Use of polymerized extracts may make several years of protection possible following a single series of fifteen weekly injections.

The peak flowmeter has proved to be an excellent device in enlisting patients and their families as active associates with their physicians in managing asthma. Some experts see the day when personal computers will play a similar role as they will share information between patient and doctor regarding symptoms and treatment.

Dr. Sly was even willing to say that prevention, as well as control of asthma, may be possible through modifications in lifestyle, diet, avoidance of irritants and allergens, better drugs, and injection treatment. There is light at the end of the tunnel!

CHAPTER

15

✿ ✿ ✿

Success Stories:
From Falstaff to
Kenny Rogers

✿✿

I'm physically and emotionally repulsed by the idea that the patient causes asthma psychologically.

—PAMELA

For many years the general public has viewed asthma more as a character defect than a disease. The difficulty in determining triggers, the rapidity with which some attacks develop, and the chronic nature of the disease are in part responsible for the misconception that asthma is largely self-induced. Frequently asthma is dismissed with disdain or derision by misinformed adults, making the management of this frustrating disease even more difficult. This theory is not just wrong but it is cruel. Because of this erroneous perception, many young asthmatics, in addition to their disease, must also carry the burden of guilt for having a condition they can't easily control.

Unfortunately, the all-too-common portrait of asthmatics in film and literature is that of a sickly and frail individual confined to a sedentary lifestyle devoid of strenuous exercise. Fortunately, my parents never let this type of stereotype influence our home life. Instead, they gave me the confidence to defy such stereotypes, thus enabling me to do such things as travel and camp throughout the United States, live and travel abroad, live and work on farms, use a bicycle as my main form of transportation for years, and take a career that finds me outside almost year-round.

—DAVID

Books, plays, and movies, from Shakespeare to Woody Allen, have presented the asthmatic as a ridiculous wimp, avoiding responsibility by self-induced wheezing. The wheezing buffoon, Falstaff, is a character in many of Shakespeare's plays, usually disregarding duty for debauchery. In melodramas the devious landlord is often depicted as a wheezing weakling. Neil Simon's play *The Odd Couple* gives us Felix Unger, a notorious hypochondriac, spontaneously wheezing when situations become difficult.

In Woody Allen's movie *Hannah and Her Sisters*, Allen plays a character who exhibits episodes of asthma and allergy in direct relationship to his feelings of inadequacy and discontent. His wheezing disappears as his personal life improves. *Dead Poets Society* portrays one of the boys at the boarding school as an asthmatic nerd, bossed around by his overbearing father and constantly blowing his nose. He is the last of the students to stand up on his desk in salute to Robin Williams as he departs—a supposed comment on his lack of innate courage.

These characters, and the situations they find themselves in, are amusing, interesting, and entertaining, but they are pure fiction. In real life asthmatics don't run from adversity. They must confront it each time they have an attack.

The most important skill to master on the way to maturity is self-discipline. In coping with the many restrictions imposed by their disease, asthmatic children must learn this skill earlier than their peers. It's essential in fighting the daily battle with their illness. Perhaps it is one of the reasons many asthmatics have reached prominence in competitive fields as adults.

Five U.S. swimmers who have won Olympic gold medals have had asthma. Nancy Hogshead, winner of three gold medals and one silver in the 1984 Olympics, wrote a book on asthma and exercise (see Reading List at the end of this book). Greg Louganis, the 1984 Olympic diving gold medalist, got his start in the pool for asthma therapy. Jackie Joyner-Kersee, national and international champion in track and field, has asthma. Danny Manning, 1987–88 NCAA Basketball Player of the Year, does too, along with Bill Koch, top cross-country ski racer.

Chet Atkins, who plays the guitar with consummate skill, and commands the respect and awe of the musical community, spent many hours practicing when asthma limited more strenuous activities. Kenny Rogers has followed in this tradition, and is one of the most popular singers and guitar players in the country. He, too, developed his many talents while overcoming childhood asthma.

Asthmatics' capacity to excel extends as well to politics. Robert Mosbacher, secretary of commerce, is a member of the asthmatics club. One of the most sought-after and prestigious honors in the field of literature and journalism is the Pulitzer Prize. Joseph Pulitzer envisioned and endowed this award. He was an asthmatic. And I think the answer to the enigma of why Napoleon posed with his hand inside his tunic is explained by the fact that he had asthma. He was counting intakes of breath!

> *Asthma is a very difficult disease to grow up with. It is also hard to explain the fear and pain of an asthma attack. You must experience it yourself—the tightness in your chest, the light-headedness, the nausea, the feeling of suffocation. The fear you will die and the secret hope that in dying you will be relieved of your pain.*
>
> *—MELISSA*

Most of us never think about breathing. We take it for granted. For thousands of children, periodic asthma attacks make breathing the hardest thing they'll ever do. If you have ever been caught under the waves at the ocean, you may have experienced the frightening feeling of suffocation well known to the asthmatic. The most important success story for most childhood asthmatics is overcoming their illness and preparing themselves to lead full, productive lives. We can help our children make this transition sooner by understanding and meeting their medical and emotional needs.

Raising children is a balancing act, and most parents have to learn the intricacies as they go along. We've learned a lot from our children. When I look back on the times asthma restricted them to bedrest, I remember their ingenuity. David loved small replicas of red-coated English soldiers. Like the Robert Louis Stevenson poem, "The Land of Counterpane," those soldiers marched up and down the bed covers, and David was not deterred when a coughing spasm decimated the ranks. Melissa created fashions out of facial tissues for Barbie and her friends. And Pamela, as a class officer, directed and organized her entire class by phone. They never let the physical manifestations of asthma interfere with their intellect or spirit. We've tried hard to follow their lead.

Asthma has always been a part of my life, of my family. Asthma has seldom, however, been a part of my daily thoughts or fears. The main force in relieving any inhibitions that asthma may have levied on my lifestyle has been my parents, who never told me what I couldn't do, but used their energy to support me in whatever endeavors I decided to undertake. It is in large part due to this unshakable support that asthma never has become a word that means "you can't do that," or "you have to settle for this." Instead, I see asthma simply as a condition that makes life a bit more challenging.

—DAVID

APPENDIX: Accredited Programs in Allergy/Immunology

Experts in allergic diseases reside at the following hospitals, clinics, and medical centers. They may be able to help solve asthma problems that are beyond the experience of local physicians.

California

LA JOLLA

Scripps Clinic and Research Foundation Program
Scripps Clinic and Research Foundation
Program Director:
Ronald A Simon, MD
David A Mathison, MD
Scripps Clinic and Research Foundation
10666 N Torrey Pines Rd
La Jolla CA 92037
Length: 2 Year(s); **Total Positions:** 2
OPV-P 0; OPV-A 0; OPV-M 5,000; OPV-CI 400
Program ID# 0200531002

LOS ANGELES

Childrens Hospital of Los Angeles Program
Childrens Hospital of Los Angeles
Program Director:
Joseph A Church, MD
Childrens Hospital of Los Angeles
4650 Sunset Blvd
Los Angeles CA 90027
Length: 2 Year(s); **Total Positions:** 2
OPV-P 5,000; OPV-A 500; OPV-M 500; OPV-CI 500
Program ID# 0200521049

Kaiser Permanente Medical Center Los Angeles Program
Kaiser Foundation Hospital (Los Angeles)

▶**Information Not Provided** *Shared-Schedule Positions Available*
OPV-P = *Outpatient Visits Pediatric;* **OPV-A** = *Outpatient Visits Adult;* **OPV-M** = *Outpatient Visits Mixed;* **OPV-CI** = *Clinical Immunology*

Program Director:
Michael Kaplan, MD
Kaiser Foundation Hospital
4867 Sunset Boulevard
Los Angeles CA 90027
Length: 2 Year(s); **Total Positions:** 2
OPV-P 0; OPV-A 0; OPV-M 10,000;
OPV-CI 450
Program ID# 0200512003

U C L A Hospital and Clinics, Center for The Health Sciences Program
U C L A Medical Center
Program Director:
E Richard Stiehm, MD
Andrew Saxon, MD
U C L A Center for the Health Sciences
Dept of Allergy/Immunology
Los Angeles CA 90024
Length: 2 Year(s); **Total Positions:** 9
OPV-P 2,620; OPV-A 1,200; OPV-M 4,220; OPV-CI 400
Program ID# 0200511038

West Los Angeles Veterans Administration Medical Center (Wadsworth Division) Program
Veterans Administration Medical Center (Wadsworth)
Program Director:
William B Klaustermeyer, MD
West Los Angeles Veterans Admin Med Ctr (Wadsworth Div)
Allergy/Immunology Section
W111r
Los Angeles CA 90073
Length: 2 Year(s); **Total Positions:** 2
OPV-P 1,200; OPV-A 4,600; OPV-M 400; OPV-CI 200
Program ID # 0200521096

▶**University of Southern California Program**
Los Angeles County-U S C Medical Center
Program Director:
Zack H Haddad, MD
Los Angeles County-U S C Medical Center
1129 N State. ST
Los Angeles CA 90033
Length: 2 Year(s); **Total Positions:** 0
OPV-P 0; OPV-A 0; OPV-M 0; OPV-CI 0
Program ID# 0200521065

ORANGE
University of California (Irvine) Program
University of California Irvine Medical Center
Veterans Administration Medical Center (Long Beach)
Program Director:
Sudhir Gupta, MD
Univ of Caifornia, Irvine
Medical Sciences I, C264a
Irvine CA 92717
Length: 2 Year(s); **Total Positions:** 2
OPV-P 1,955; OPV-A 2,420; OPV-M 0; OPV-CI 300
Program ID# 0200521064

SACRAMENTO
University of California (Davis) Program ★
Univ of California (Davis) Medical Center (Sacramento)
Program Director:
M Eric Gershwin, MD
School of Medicine, Sect Rheumatology-Allergy, T B 192
Univ of California (Davis)
Davis CA 95616

Length: 2 Year(s); **Total Positions:** 2
OPV-P 0; OPV-A 0; OPV-M 1,200;
OPV-CI 1,200
Program ID# 0200521048

SAN DIEGO
University of California (San Diego) Program
U C S D Medical Center
Program Director:
Robert N Hamburger, MD
Stephen I Wasserman, MD
School of Medicine, Division of
Allergic & Immunologic Dis
U C S D Medical Center
San Diego CA 92103
Length: 2 Year(s); **Total Positions:** 2
OPV-P 800; OPV-A 0; OPV-M
4,000; OPV-CI 60
Program ID# 0200521966

SAN FRANCISCO
University of California (San Francisco) Program
Medical Center at the Univ of
California San Francisco
Program Director:
Oscar L Frick, MD
Edward J Goetzl, MD
Univ of Calfiornia, San Francisco
Dept of Medicine U-332
San Francisco CA 94143
Length: 2 Year(s); **Total Positions:** 6
OPV-P 1,200; OPV-A 0; OPV-M
480; OPV-CI 400
Program ID# 0200521059

STANFORD
Stanford University Program
Stanford University Hospital
Program Director:
Norman J Lewiston, MD

Children's Hospital At Stanford
520 Willow Rd
Palo Alto CA 94304
Length: 2 Year(s); **Total Positions:** 4
OPV-P 1,600; OPV-A 700; OPV-M
0; OPV-CI 200
Program ID# 0200521006

TORRANCE
Los Angeles County-Harbor-U C L A Medical Center Program
Los Angeles County-Harbor-
U C L A Medical Center
Program Director:
Gildon Beall, MD
Douglas C Heiner, MD
Los Angeles County-Harbor-
UCLA Medical Center
1000 W Carson St
Torrance CA 90509
Length: 2 Year(s); **Total Positions:** 4
OPV-P 0; OPV-A 0; OPV-M 0;
OPV-CI 0
Program ID# 0200521102

Colorado

AURORA
Fitzsimons Army Medical Center Program
Fitzsimons Army Medical Center
Program Director:
Col Richard W Weber, MD
Fitzsimons Army Medical Center, Allergy and Immunology
Service
Aurora CO 80045
Length: 2 Year(s); **Total Positions:** 7
OPV-P 2,900; OPV-A 6,200; OPV-M 0; OPV-CI 50
Program ID# 0200721067

DENVER
University of Colorado Program A
University of Colorado Health
Sciences Center
National Jewish Ctr for Immu-
nology and Respiratory Medi-
cine
Program Director:
Stanley J Szetler, MD
National Jewish Center for Im-
munology and Respiratory
Med
1400 Jackson St
Denver CO 80206
Length: 2 Year(s); **Total Posi-
tions:** 15
OPV-P 2,153; OPV-A 4,113; OPV-
M 6,276; OPV-CI 178
Program ID# 0200731010

▶University of Colorado
Program B
University of Colorado Health
Sciences Center
National Jewish Ctr for Immu-
nology and Respiratory Medi-
cine
Program Director:
Harold S Nelson, MD
Henry N Claman, MD
University of Colorado School
of Medicine
4200 E Ninth Ave
Denver CO 80262
Length: 2 Year(s); **Total Posi-
tions:** 9
OPV-P 2,600; OPV-A 6,000; OPV-
M 0; OPV-CI 750
Program ID# 0200731086

Connecticut

NEW HAVEN
**Yale-New Haven Medical Center
Program**

Yale-New Haven Hospital
Program Director:
Philip W Askenase, MD
Yale-New Haven Hospital
20 York Street
New Haven CT 06504
Length: 2 Year(s); **Total Posi-
tions:** 3
OPV-P 0; OPV-A 0; OPV-M 0;
OPV-CI 0
Program ID# 0200821099

D.C.

WASHINGTON
**Children's Hospital National
Medical Center Program**
Children's Hospital National
Medical Center
Program Director:
R Michael Sly, MD
Children's Hospital National
Medical Center
111 Michigan Ave, N W
Washington DC 20010
Length: 2 Year(s); **Total Posi-
tions:** 2
OPV-P 4,400; OPV-A 1,650; OPV-
M 0; OPV-CI 450
Program ID# 0201011039

Georgetown University Program
Georgetown University Hospital
Program Director:
Jospeh A Bellanti, MD
Robert T Scanlon, MD
Georgetown University Hospital
3800 Reservoir Rd, N W
Washington DC 20007
Length: 2 Year(s); **Total Posi-
tions:** 4
OPV-P 0; OPV-A 0; OPV-M 0;
OPV-CI 0
Program ID# 0201021011

Howard University Program
  Howard University Hospital
  District of Columbia General
  Hospital
Program Director:
  Sheryl E Lucas, MD
  Howard University Hospital
  2041 Georgia Ave, N W
  Washington DC 20060
Length: 2 Year(s); **Total Positions:** 2
OPV-P 1,913; OPV-A 720; OPV-M 0; OPV-CI 120
Program ID# 0201021068

Walter Reed Army Medical Center Program
Program Director:
  Lt Col Gary B Carpenter, MD
  Walter Reed Army Medical Center
  Allergy/Immunology Service
  Washington DC 20307
Length: 2 Year(s); **Total Positions:** 7
OPV-P 0; OPV-A 0; OPV-M 21,900; OPV-CI 310
Program ID# 0201011087

Florida

ST PETERSBURG
University of South Florida Program
  All Children's Hospital-Univ of South Florida Coll of Med
Program Director:
  Robert A Good, Ph D,MD
  All Children's Hospital, Clinical Immunology & Allergy
  801 Sixth Street South
  St Petersburg FL 33701
Length: 2 Year(s); **Total Positions:** 5
Program ID# 0201121106

TAMPA
University of South Florida Program
  James A Haley Veterans Hospital
  University of South Florida Medical Clinics
Program Director:
  Richard F Lockey, MD
  James A Haley Veterans Hospital
  13000 Bruce B Downs Blvd
  (Var 111d)
  Tampa FL 33612
Length: 2 Year(s); **Total Positions:** 3
OPV-P 1,000; OPV-A 3,000; OPV-M 6,000; OPV-CI 600
Program ID# 0201121093

Georgia

ATLANTA
Emory University Program
  Henrietta Egleston Hospital for Children
  Grady Memorial Hospital
Program Director:
  Thomas F Smith, MD
  Dept of Pediatrics
  69 Butler St, S E
  Atlanta GA 30303
Length: 2 Year(s); **Total Positions:** 3
OPV-P 1,500; OPV-A 900; OPV-M 300; OPV-CI 900
Program ID# 0201221101

AUGUSTA
Medical College of Georgia Program
  Medical College of Georgia Hospital and Clinics

Program Director:
Betty B Wray, MD
Dept of Pediatrics and Medicine
Med Coll of Georgia, C J 141
Augusta GA 30912
Length: 2 Year(s); **Total Positions:** 3
OPV-P 0; OPV-A 0; OPV-M 7,400; OPV-CI 1,000
Program ID# 0201221013

Illinois

CHICAGO
Northwestern University Medical School Program
Northwestern Memorial Hospital
Children's Memorial Hospital
Program Director:
Roy Patterson, MD
Northwestern University Medical School
303 E Chicago Ave
Chicago IL 60611
Length: 2 Year(s); **Total Positions:** 7
OPV-P 3,550; OPV-A 0; OPV-M 21,000; OPV-CI 1,700
Program ID# 0201631016

Rush-Presbyterian-St Luke's Medical Center Program
Rush-Presbyterian-St Luke's Medical Center
Program Director:
Howard J Zeitz, MD
Rush-Presbyterian-St Luke's Medical Center
1753 W Congress Pkwy
Chicago IL 60612
Length: 2 Year(s); **Total Positions:** 4
OPV-P 0; OPV-A 0; OPV-M 6,500; OPV-CI 2,500

Program ID# 0201621044

▶**Grant Hospital of Chicago Program**
Grant Hospital of Chicago
Program Director:
Howard J Zeitz, MD
Grant Hospital of Chicago
550 W Webster Ave
Chicago IL 60614
Length: 2 Year(s); **Total Positions:** 2
OPV-P 0; OPV-A 0; OPV-M 3,000; OPV-CI 1,000
Program ID# 0201612015

Iowa

IOWA CITY
University of Iowa Hospitals and Clinics Program A
University of Iowa Hospitals and Clinics
Program Director:
Miles Weinberger, MD
University of Iowa Hospital and Clinics
Dept of Pediatrics
Iowa City IA 52242
Length: 2 Year(s); **Total Positions:** 3
OPV-P 1,500; OPV-A 2,500; OPV-M 1,500; OPV-CI 1,500
Program ID# 0201821080

University of Iowa Hospitals and Clinics Program B
University of Iowa Hospitals and Clinics
Program Director:
Hal B Richerson, MD
University of Iowa Hospitals and Clinics
Dept of Internal Medicine
Iowa City IA 52242

Length: 2 Year(s); **Total Positions:** 4
OPV-P 0; OPV-A 2,424; OPV-M 100; OPV-CI 450
Program ID# 0201821081

Kansas

KANSAS CITY
University of Kansas Medical Center/Children's Mercy Hospital Program
University of Kansas Medical Center
Children's Mercy Hospital
Program Director:
Daniel J Stechschulte, MD
University of Kansas Medical Center, Div Allergy/ Immunology
39th and Rainbow
Kansas City KS 66103
Length: 2 Year(s); **Total Positions:** 4
OPV-P 10,500; OPV-A 3,500; OPV-M 0; OPV-CI 500
Program ID# 0201921030

Kentucky

LOUISVILLE
University of Louisville Program
Humana Hospital-University of Louisville
Kosair Children's Hospital
Norton Hospital
Program Director:
John M Karibo, MD
Hobert L Pence, MD
464 Medical Towers South
Louisville KY 40202
Length: 2 Year(s); **Total Positions:** 2
OPV-P 1,490; OPV-A 472; OPV-M 1,892; OPV-CI 156

Program ID# 0202021050

Louisiana

NEW ORLEANS
Charity Hospital of Louisiana-L S U Division Program
Charity Hospital of Louisiana-L S U Division
Program Director:
John Strimus, MD
Prem Kumar, MD
L S U School of Medicine, Allergy/Immunology Service
1542 Tulane Ave
New Orleans LA 70112
Length: 2 Year(s); **Total Positions:** 4
OPV-P 2,912; OPV-A 1,362; OPV-M 443; OPV-CI 371
Program ID# 0202121070

Tulane University Program
Tulane Medical Center Hospital
Charity Hospital of Louisiana-Tulane Division
Veterans Admin Med Center-Tulane Service (New Orleans)
Program Director:
John E Salvaggio, MD
Tulane Medical Center, Section of Allergy/Immunology
1430 Tulane Ave
New Orleans LA 70112
Length: 2 Year(s); **Total Positions:** 3
OPV-P 1,000; OPV-A 1,000; OPV-M 0; OPV-CI 500
Program ID# 0202131017

SHREVEPORT
Louisiana State University (Shreveport) Program
Louisiana State University Hospital

Program Director:
Bettina C Hilman, MD
Louisiana State University Hospital
P O Box 33932
Shreveport LA 71130
Length: 2 Year(s); **Total Positions:** 3
OPV-P 26,048; OPV-A 413; OPV-M 1,346; OPV-CI 0
Program ID# 0202121060

Maryland

BALTIMORE
Johns Hopkins University Program
Good Samaritan Hospital of Maryland
Johns Hopkins Hospital
Program Director:
Philip S Norman, MD
Peyton A Eggleston, MD
Johns Hopkins University
School of Medicine
5601 Loch Raven Blvd
Baltimore, MD 21239
Length: 2 Year(s); **Total Positions:** 10
OPV-P 1,600; OPV-A 4,000; OPV-M 0; OPV-CI 230
Program ID# 0202321094

BETHESDA
National Institutes of Health Warren Grant Magnuson Clinical Center Program
N I H Warren Grant Magnuson Clinical Center
Program Director:
Michael A Kaliner, MD
National Institutes of Health
Clinical Ctr, Building 10
Room 11 C 205
Bethesda MD 20892

Length: 2 Year(s); **Total Positions:** 12
OPV-P 500; OPV-A 2,000; OPV-M 0; OPV-CI 500
Program ID# 0202321090

Massachusetts

BOSTON
Brigham and Women's Hospital Program
Brigham and Women's Hospital
Program Director:
Albert L Sheffer, MD
Brigham and Women's Hospital
110 Francis St
Boston MA 02215
Length: 2 Year(s); **Total Positions:** 4
OPV-P 5,100; OPV-A 375; OPV-M 4,800; OPV-CI 1,450
Program ID# 0202421031

Massachusetts General Hospital Program
Massachusetts General Hospital
Program Director:
Kurt J Bloch, MD
Massachusetts General Hospital
Fruit St
Boston MA 02114
Length: 2 Year(s); **Total Positions:** 2
OPV-P 250; OPV-A 5,000; OPV-M 0; OPV-CI 200
Program ID# 0202421051

New England Medical Center Hospitals Program
New England Medical Center Hospitals
Program Director:
Lanny J Rosenwasser, MD
New England Medical Center
171 Harrison Ave, Box 30
Boston MA 02111

Length: 2 Year(s); **Total Positions:** 4
OPV-P 1,080; OPV-A 2,100; OPV-M 0; OPV-CI 2,311
Program ID# 0202421052

▶**Children's Hospital Program**
Children's Hospital
Program Director:
Raif S Geha, MD
Children's Hospital
300 Longwood Ave
Boston MA 02115
Length: 2 Year(s); **Total Positions:** 0
OPV-P 6,000; OPV-A 500; OPV-M 0; OPV-CI 100
Program ID# 0202421061

Michigan

ANN ARBOR
University of Michigan Program
University of Michigan Hospitals
Program Director:
William R Solomon, MD
Univ of Michigan Hospitals, Allergy Division
3918 Taubman Center
Ann Arbor MI 48109
Length: 2 Year(s); **Total Positions:** 4
OPV-P 0; OPV-A 0; OPV-M 5,218; OPV-CI 200
Program ID# 0202521045

DETROIT
Henry Ford Hospital Program
Henry Ford Hospital
Program Director:
John A Anderson, MD
Henry Ford Hospital
2799 W Grand Blvd
Detroit MI 48202

Length: 2 Year(s); **Total Positions:** 4
OPV-P 8,000; OPV-A 12,000; OPV-M 0; OPV-CI 1,000
Program ID# 0202511032

Wayne State University Program
Children's Hospital of Michigan
Detroit Receiving Hospital and University Health Center
Harper-Grace Hospitals-Harper Division
Program Director:
Helen A Papaioanou, MD
Children's Hospital of Michigan
3901 Beaubien Blvd
Detroit MI 48201
Length: 2 Year(s); **Total Positions:** 2
OPV-P 4,650; OPV-A 2,700; OPV-M 0; OPV-CI 1,500
Program ID# 0202521071

Minnesota

MINNEAPOLIS
University of Minnesota Program
University of Minnesota Hospital and Clinic
Program Director:
M N Blumenthal, MD
Univ of Minnesota, Box 434
U M H C
420 Delaware St
Minneapolis MN 55455
Length: 2 Year(s); **Total Positions:** 2
OPV-P 1,200; OPV-A 2,950; OPV-M 5,300; OPV-CI 1,000
Program ID# 0202621091

ROCHESTER
Mayo Graduate School of Medicine Program A

Mayo Graduate School of
Medicine-Mayo Clinic
Rochester Methodist Hospital
Program Director:
Charles E Reed, MD
Mayo Graduate School of Medicine
200 First St, S W
Rochester MN 55905
Length: 2 Year(s); **Total Positions:** 4
OPV-P 0; OPV-A 0; OPV-M 13,000;
OPV-CI 0
Program ID# 0202611018

Mayo Graduate School of Medicine Program B
Mayo Graduate School of
Medicine-Mayo Clinic
St Marys Hospital of Rochester
Program Director:
Edward J O'Connell, MD
John W Yunginger, MD
Mayo Graduate School of Medicine
200 First St, S W
Rochester MN 55905
Length: 2 Year(s); **Total Positions:** 2
OPV-P 3,235; OPV-A 15,582; OPV-M 0; OPV-CI 0
Program ID# 0202621057

Missouri

ST LOUIS
St Louis University Group of Hospitals Program
University Hospital-St Louis
University Medical Center
Cardinal Glennon Children's
Hospital
Program Director:
Raymond G Slavin, MD
St Louis University School of
Medicine

1402 S Grand
St Louis MO 63104
Length: 2 Year(s); **Total Positions:** 3
OPV-P 1,325; OPV-A 3,300; OPV-M 1,600; OPV-CI 50
Program ID# 0202821019

Washington University School of Medicine Program
Washington University School
of Medicine
Barnes Hospital
Jewish Hospital of St Louis At
Washington Univ Med Ctr
St Louis Children's Hospital
Program Director:
H James Wedner, MD
Washington University School
of Medicine
660 E Euclid
St Louis MO 63110
Length: 2 Year(s); **Total Positions:** 3
OPV-P 1,175; OPV-A 5,566; OPV-M 0; OPV-CI 7,222
Program ID# 0202821095

Nebraska

OMAHA
Creighton University Program
St Joseph Hospital
Program Director:
Robert G Townley, MD
Creighton University School of
Medicine
2500 California St
Omaha NE 68178
Length: 2 Year(s); **Total Positions:** 3
OPV-P 2,000; OPV-A 6,980; OPV-M 8,380; OPV-CI 2,900
Program ID# 0203021088

New Jersey

NEWARK

U M D N J-New Jersey Medical School Program
Childrens Hospital of New Jersey (United Hospitals Med Ctr)
U M D N J-University Hospital
Veterans Administration Medical Center (East Orange)
Program Director:
James M Oleske, MD
U M D N J-New Jersey Medical School
185 South Orange Avenue
Newark NJ 07103
Length: 2 Year(s); **Total Positions:** 3
OPV-P 800; OPV-A 500; OPV-M 1,000; OPV-CI 1,200
Program ID# 0203311040

New York

BRONX

Albert Einstein College of Medicine Program
Bronx Municipal Hospital Center
Jack D Weiler Hospital of Albert Einstein Coll of Medicine
Program Director:
Arye Rubinstein, MD
Albert Einstein College of Medicine
1300 Morris Park Ave
New York (Bronx) NY 10461
Length: 2 Year(s); **Total Positions:** 6
OPV-P 0; OPV-A 860; OPV-M 480; OPV-CI 800
Program ID# 0203521054

BROOKLYN

Long Island College Hospital Program
Long Island College Hospital
Program Director:
Lawrence T Chiaramonte, MD
Long Island College Hospital
340 Henry St
Brooklyn NY 11201
Length: 2 Year(s); **Total Positions:** 5
OPV-P 3,397; OPV-A 4,048; OPV-M 1,613; OPV-CI 107
Program ID# 0203511041

S U N Y Health Science Center At Brooklyn Program ✶
University Hospital-S U N Y Health Science Ctr At Brooklyn
Kings County Hospital Center
Program Director:
Alan S Josephson, MD
Downstate Medical Center
450 Clarkson Ave
Brooklyn NY 11203
Length: 2 Year(s); **Total Positions:** 3
OPV-P 0; OPV-A 0; OPV-M 3,750; OPV-CI 250
Program ID# 0203521092

BUFFALO

State University of New York At Buffalo Graduate Medical-Dental Education Consortium Program
Buffalo General Hospital Corp
Children's Hospital of Buffalo
Program Director:
Elliott Middleton Jr. MD
Buffalo General Hospital
100 High St
Buffalo NY 14203
Length: 2 Year(s); **Total Positions:** 4

OPV-P 2,649; OPV-A 1,343; OPV-M 0; OPV-CI 190
Program ID# 0203521053

EAST MEADOW
Nassau County Medical Center Program
Nassau County Medical Center
North Shore University Hospital
Program Director:
Marianne Frieri, PhD, MD
Nassau County Medical Center, Dept of Allergy and Immunology
2201 Hempstead Turnpike
East Meadow NY 11554
Length: 2 Year(s); **Total Positions:** 4
OPV-P 1,231; OPV-A 1,155; OPV-M 0; OPV-CI 1,515
Program ID# 0203511020

NEW HYDE PARK
Long Island Jewish Medical Center Program
Schneider Children's Hosp (Long Island Jewish Med Ctr)
Program Director:
Vincent R Bonagura, MD
Long Island Jewish Medical Center
New Hyde Park NY 11042
Length: 2 Year(s); **Total Positions:** 0
Program ID# 0203521105

NEW YORK
Mount Sinai School, of Medicine Program
Mount Sinai Hospital
Program Director:
Joseph M Hasser, MD
Mount Sinai Hospital
One Gustave L Levy Pl
New York NY 10029

Length: 2 Year(s); **Total Positions:** 4
OPV-P 800; OPV-A 5,500; OPV-M 0; OPV-CI 1,000
Program ID# 0203521083

New York Hospital/Cornell Medical Center Program A
New York Hospital
Program Director:
Irwin Rappaport, MD
Ingrid K Rosner, MD
New York Hospital, Dept of Pediatrics
525 E 68th St
New York NY 10021
Length: 2 Year(s); **Total Positions:** 2
OPV-P 3,560; OPV-A 0; OPV-M 0; OPV-CI 100
Program ID# 0203521046

New York Hospital/Cornell Medical Center Program B
New York Hospital
Program Director:
Gregory W Siskind, MD
Cornell University Medical College
1300 York Ave
New York NY 10021
Length: 2 Year(s); **Total Positions:** 2
OPV-P 1,150; OPV-A 3,220; OPV-M 200; OPV-CI 200
Program ID# 0203521084

Presbyterian Hospital In the City of New York Program
Presbyterian Hospital in the City of New York
Program Director:
William J Davis, MD
Columbia University College of Physicians and Surgeons
630 W 168th St

New York NY 10032
Length: 2 Year(s); **Total Positions:** 2
OPV-P 3,200; OPV-A 1,500; OPV-M 0; OPV-CI 450
Program ID# 0203521082

St Luke's-Roosevelt Hospital Center Program
St Luke's-Roosevelt Hospital Center-Roosevelt Division
Program Director:
Michael H Grieco, MD
R A Cooke Institute of Allergy
428 West 59th St
New York NY 10019
Length: 2 Year(s); **Total Positions:** 3
OPV-P 900; OPV-A 7,900; OPV-M 8,800; OPV-CI 600
Program ID# 0203511042

ROCHESTER
University of Rochester Program
Strong Memorial Hospital of the University of Rochester
Program Director:
Stephen I Rosenfeld, MD
Strong Memorial Hospital
601 Elmwood Ave, Box 695
Rochester NY 14642
Length: 2 Year(s); **Total Positions:** 3
OPV-P 2,500; OPV-A 4,500; OPV-M 3,600; OPV-CI 1,600
Program ID# 0203511043

STONY BROOK
S U N Y At Stony Brook Program
University Hospital-S U N Y At Stony Brook
Veterans Administration Medical Center (Northport)
Program Director:
Peter Gorevic, MD

Div of Allergy/Rheumatology,
Clinical Immunology
S U N Y Health Sciences Center
Stony Brook NY 11794
Length: 2 Year(s); **Total Positions:** 4
OPV-P 12; OPV-A 350; OPV-M 8,000; OPV-CI 0
Program ID# 0203521089

North Carolina

DURHAM
Duke University Medical Center Program
Duke University Medical Center
Program Director:
Rebecca Buckley, MD
Duke University Medical Center
Div Ped Allergy/Immunology
Box 2898
Durham NC 27710
Length: 2 Year(s); **Total Positions:** 9
OPV-P 21,500; OPV-A 87,500; OPV-M 0; OPV-CI 5,000
Program ID# 0203621022

WINSTON-SALEM
Bowman Gray School of Medicine Program
North Carolina Baptist Hospital
Program Director:
John W Georgitis, MD
Bowman Gray School of Medicine
300 S Hawthorne
Winston-Salem NC 27103
Length: 2 Year(s); **Total Positions:** 2
OPV-P 2,500; OPV-A 100; OPV-M 0; OPV-CI 50
Program ID# 0203611047

OHIO

CINCINNATI

University of Cincinnati Hospital Group Program B
Children's Hospital Medical Center
University of Cincinnati Hospital
Program Director:
Thomas J Fischer, MD
Children's Hospital Medical Center
Elland and Bethesda Aves
Cincinnati OH 45229
Length: 2 Year(s); **Total Positions:** 2
OPV-P 1,155; OPV-A 0; OPV-M 0; OPV-CI 8,744
Program ID# 0203821033

▶**University of Cincinnati Hospital Group Program A**
University of Cincinnati Hospital
Veterans Administration Medical Center (Cincinnati)
Program Director:
I Leonard Bernstein, MD
David I Bernstein, MD
University of Cincinnati Medical Center
Mail Location 563
Cincinnati OH 45267
Length: 2 Year(s); **Total Positions:** 0
OPV-P 5,050; OPV-A 6,500; OPV-M 3,000; OPV-CI 8,000
Program ID# 0203821072

CLEVELAND

Cleveland Clinic Foundation Program
Cleveland Clinic Foundation
Program Director:
Sami L Bahna, MD

Cleveland Clinic Foundation, Allergy & Immunology
9500 Euclid Avenue
Cleveland OH 44106
Length: 2 Year(s); **Total Positions:** 2
OPV-P 0; OPV-A 0; OPV-M 0; OPV-CI 0
Program ID# 0203821104

Pennsylvania

PHILADELPHIA

St Christopher's Hospital for Children Program
St Christopher's Hospital for Children
Program Director:
Edward W Hein, MD
St Christopher's Hospital for Children
Fifth St and Lehigh Ave
Philadelphia PA 19133
Length: 2 Year(s); **Total Positions:** 2
OPV-P 3,650; OPV-A 3,200; OPV-M 0; OPV-CI 800
Program ID# 020412073

Thomas Jefferson University Program
Thomas Jefferson University Hospital
Program Director:
Herbert C Mansmann, Jr. MD
Jefferson Medical College
1025 Walnut St
Philadelphia PA 19107
Length: 2 Year(s); **Total Positions:** 6
OPV-P 1,362; OPV-A 5,040; OPV-M 6,402; OPV-CI 148
Program ID# 0204111034

University of Pennsylvania Program B

Children's Hospital of Philadelphia
Program Director:
Steven D Douglas, MD
Children's Hospital of Philadelphia
34th and Civic Blvd
Philadelphia PA 19104
Length: 2 Year(s); **Total Positions:** 4
OPV-P 2,900; OPV-A 4,800; OPV-M 7,700; OPV-CI 975
Program ID# 0204121074

University of Pennsylvania Program A
Hospital of the University of Pennsylvania
Program Director:
Burton Zweiman, MD
Univ of Pennsylvania School of Medicine
512 Johnson Pavillion
Philadelphia PA 19104
Length: 2 Year(s); **Total Positions:** 2
OPV-P 0; OPV-A 10,000; OPV-M 50; OPV-CI 1,000
Program ID# 0204121075

PITTSBURGH
Hospitals of the University Health Center Of Pittsburgh Program
Children's Hospital of Pittsburgh
Program Director:
Philip Fireman, MD
Children's Hospital of Pittsburgh
3705 Fifth Ave At de Soto St
Pittsburgh PA 15213
Length: 2 Year(s); **Total Positions:** 2
OPV-P 7,121; OPV-A 1,236; OPV-M 0; OPV-CI 266

Program ID# 0204121076

Rhode Island

PROVIDENCE
Rhode Island Hospital Program
Rhode Island Hospital
Program Director:
Donald E Klein, MD
Guy A Settipane, MD
Rhode Island Hospital, Dept of Medicine/Pediatrics
593 Eddy St
Providence RI 02902
Length: 2 Year(s); **Total Positions:** 2
OPV-P 1,015; OPV-A 2,573; OPV-M 3,588; OPV-CI 0
Program ID# 0204321024

Tennessee

MEMPHIS
University of Tennessee Program
LeBonheur Children's Medical Center
Baptist Memorial Hospital
Univ of Tennessee Medical Center-Wm F Bowld Hospital
Veterans Administration Medical Center (Memphis)
Program Director:
Tai-June Yoo, MD
Henry G Herrod, MD
Univ of Tennessee Coll of Med, Sect of Allergy/Immunology
956 Court Ave
Memphis TN 38163
Length: 2 Year(s); **Total Positions:** 4
OPV-P 11,000; OPV-A 2,750; OPV-M 0; OPV-CI 226
Program ID# 0204721025

NASHVILLE
Vanderbilt University Program
Vanderbilt University Medical Center
Program Director:
Samuel R Marney, MD
2501 the Vanderbilt Clinic
Dept of Allergy/Immunology
Nashville TN 37232
Length: 2 Year(s); **Total Positions:** 2
OPV-P 195; OPV-A 10,940; OPV-M 0; OPV-CI 0
Program ID# 0204721097

Texas

DALLAS
University of Texas Southwestern Medical School Program
Dallas County Hospital District-Parkland Memorial Hospital
Children's Medical Center of Dallas
Program Director:
Timothy J Sullivan, MD
Univ of Texas Health Science Center
5323 Harry Hines Blvd
Dallas TX 75235
Length: 2 Year(s); **Total Positions:** 4
OPV-P 800; OPV-A 2,200; OPV-M 50; OPV-CI 250
Program ID# 0204821085

GALVESTON
University of Texas Medical Branch Hospitals Program A
University of Texas Medical Branch Hospitals
Program Director:
J Andrew Grant, MD
University of Texas Medical Branch Hospitals

Clinical Science Bldg, Rm 409
Galveston TX 77550
Length: 2 Year(s); **Total Positions:** 4
OPV-P 1,200; OPV-A 900; OPV-M 0; OPV-CI 950
Program ID# 0204811026

University of Texas Medical Branch Hospitals Program B
University of Texas Medical Branch Hospitals
Program Director:
Armond S. Goldman, MD
Univ of Texas Medical Branch, Dept of Pediatrics
Rm C234, Child Health Center
Galveston TX 77550
Length: 2 Year(s); **Total Positions:** 3
OPV-P 1,200; OPV-A 700; OPV-M 0; OPV-CI 470
Program ID# 0204811027

HOUSTON
Baylor College of Medicine Program
Texas Children's Hospital
Methodist Hospital
Program Director:
William T Shearer, MD, PhD
Baylor College of Medicine, Dept of Pediatrics
One Baylor Plaza
Houston TX 77030
Length: 2 Year(s); **Total Positions:** 6
OPV-P 1,500; OPV-A 2,800; OPV-M 2,000; OPV-CI 400
Program ID# 0204821063

SAN ANTONIO
University of Texas At San Antonio Program
Medical Center Hospital (Of Bexar County Hosp Dist)

Brady-Green Community Health Ctr (Of Bexar County Hosp Dist)
Program Director:
William T Kniker, MD
Univ of Texas At San Antonio, Dept of Pediatrics
7703 Floyd Curl Dr
San Antonio TX 78284
Length: 2 Year(s); **Total Positions:** 2
OPV-P 3,300; OPV-A 580; OPV-M 860; OPV-CI 520
Program ID# 0204831035

Wilford Hall U S A F Medical Center Program
Wilford Hall U S A F Medical Center
Program Director:
Col Michael E Martin, MD
Wilford Hall U S A F Med Ctr, Dept of Allergy/Immunology
Lackland A F B
San Antonio TX 78236
Length: 2 Year(s); **Total Positions:** 7
OPV-P 0; OPV-A 0; OPV-M 8,000; OPV-CI 1,000
Program ID# 0204821077

Virginia

CHARLOTTESVILLE
University of Virginia Program
University of Virginia Hospitals
Program Director:
Thomas A Platts-Mills, MD
George W Ward, Jr, MD
University of Virginia
Jefferson Park Ave, Box 148
Charlottesville VA 22908
Length: 2 Year(s); **Total Positions:** 4

OPV-P 397; OPV-A 1,202; OPV-M 0; OPV-CI 0
Program ID# 0205121100

RICHMOND
Virginia Commonwealth University M C V Program
Medical College of Virginia Hospital
Program Director:
Lawrence B Schwartz, MD, PhD
Medical College of Virginia
M C V Station, Box 263
Richmond VA 23298
Length: 2 Year(s); **Total Positions:** 1
OPV-P 1,400; OPV-A 2,300; OPV-M 100; OPV-CI 125
Program ID# 0205121056

Washington

SEATTLE
University of Washington Program
University Hospital
Children's Hospital and Medical Center
Harborview Medical Center
Virginia Mason Hospital
Program Director:
Paul P Van Arsdel, Jr, MD
C Warren Bierman, MD
University Hospital
1959 N E Pacific
Seattle WA 98195
Length: 2 Year(s); **Total Positions:** 4
OPV-P 2,892; OPV-A 7,445; OPV-M 0; OPV-CI 32,889
Program ID# 0205421078

Wisconsin

MADISON
University of Wisconsin Program

University of Wisconsin Hospital and Clinics
Program Director:
William W Busse, MD
University Hospital and Clinics
600 Highland Ave, Rm H6/360
Madison WI 53792
Length: 2 Year(s); **Total Positions:** 3
OPV-P 1,000; OPV-A 1,500; OPV-M 2,000; OPV-CI 250
Program ID# 0205621028

MILWAUKEE
Medical College of Wisconsin Program
Milwaukee County Medical Complex
Children's Hospital of Wisconsin
Clement J Zablocki Veterans Administration Medical Center
Program Director:
Jordan N Fink, MD
Medical College of Wisconsin
8700 W Wisconsin Ave
Milwaukee WI 53226
Length: 2 Year(s); **Total Positions:** 1
OPV-P 0; OPV-A 0; OPV-M 8,161; OPV-CI 200
Program ID# 0205631037

United States Air Force

Wilford Hall U S A F Medical Center Program
Wilford Hall U S A F Medical Center
Program Director:
Col Michael E Martin, MD
Wilford Hall U S A F Med Ctr,
Dept of Allergy/Immunology
Lackland A F B

San Antonio TX 78236
Length: 2 Year(s); **Total Positions:** 7
OPV-P 0; OPV-A 0; OPV-M 8,000; OPV-CI 1,000
Program ID# 0204821077

United States Army

Fitzsimons Army Medical Center Program
Fitzsimons Army Medical Center
Program Director:
Col Richard W Weber, MD
Fitzsimons Army Medical Center
Allergy and Immunology Service
Aurora CO 80045
Length: 2 Year(s); **Total Positions:** 7
OPV-P 2,900; OPV-A 6,200; OPV-M 0; OPV-CI 50
Program ID# 0200721067

Walter Reed Army Medical Center Program
Walter Reed Army Medical Center
Program Director:
Lt Col Gary B Carpenter, MD
Walter Reed Army Medical Center
Allergy/Immunology Service
Washington DC 20307
Length: 2 Year(s); **Total Positions:** 7
OPV-P 0; OPV-A 0; OPV-M 21,900; OPV-CI 310
Program ID# 0201011087

Federal

National Institutes of Health Warren Grant Magnuson Clinical Center Program
N I H Warren Grant Magnuson Clinical Center
Program Director:
Michael A Kaliner, MD
National Institutes of Health Clinical Ctr, Building 10
Room 11 C 205
Bethesda MD 20892
Length: 2 Year(s); **Total Positions:** 12
OPV-P 500; OPV-A 2,000; OPV-M 0; OPV-CI 500
Program ID# 0202321090

Veterans Administration

West Los Angeles Veterans Administration Medical Center (Wadsworth Division) Program
Veterans Administration Medical Center (Wadsworth)
Program Director:
William B Klaustermeyer, MD
West Los Angeles Veterans Admin Med Ctr (Wadsworth Div)
Allergy/Immunology Section
W111r
Los Angeles CA 90073
Length: 2 Year(s); **Total Positions:** 2
OPV-P 1,200; OPV-A 4,600; OPV-M 400; OPV-CI 200
Program ID# 0200521096

University of South Florida Program
James A Haley Veterans Hospital
University of South Florida Medical Clinics
Program Director:
Richard F Lockey, MD
James A Haley Veterans Hospital
13000 Bruce B Downs Blvd (Var 111d)
Tampa FL 33612
Length: 2 Year(s); **Total Positions:** 3
OPV-P 1,000; OPV-A 3,000; OPV-M 6,000; OPV-CI 600
Program ID# 0201121093

Reprinted from the Directory of Graduate and Education Programs,
1989–1990, *with kind permission from the American Medical Association.*

READING LIST

Here is a brief list of recommended books. Included are a number of pieces of fiction about young people who are dealing with asthma.

All About Asthma and How to Live With It, by Glenn H. Paul and Barbara A. Faloglia; Sterling Publishing Co., Inc., 1988.
An excellent reference guide—brief answers, charts, statistics, and illustrations on everything you ever wanted to know about asthma. Includes a section on childhood asthma.

The Allergy Self-Help Book, by Sharon Faelten and the editors of *Prevention* magazine, 1983.
Asthma is just one of the reaction diseases addressed here, along with hay fever, headaches, fatigue, skin and digestive problems. This book concentrates on behaviors and diets that can help in combating these problems.

Appointment with a Stranger, by Jean Thesman; Houghton Mifflin Co., 1989.
An exciting, well-written book about a teenaged girl who suffers chronic, and sometimes acute, asthma. Features typical high school friendships and romances, along with an occult mystery. Deals directly with the pain and embarrassment asthma can cause, but ends on an upbeat note.

Asthma, by Allan Weinstein; McGraw Hill, 1987.
Complete encyclopedia of asthma, well written and annotated by a doctor who speaks in lay terms.

Asthma and Exercise, by Nancy Hogshead; Henry Holt & Co., 1990.
From a three-gold-medal winner Olympic swimmer, this book dispels all myths about asthmatics staying away from exercise. Gives specific advice on developing aerobic exercise approaches that have been shown to improve lung capacity in asthmatics.

Asthma: Stop Suffering, Start Living, by M. Eric Gershwin and E. L. Klingelhofer; Addison-Wesley Publishing Co., 1986.
A wonderfully comprehensive and detailed book by a doctor who became a specialist because his daughter developed severe asthma. Photos illustrate methods for breathing and using medical equipment.

Breathing Exercises for Asthma, by Karen R. Butts; Charles Thomas, Publisher, 1980.
Yoga-like exercises intended to aid the lungs, breathing passages, and glands to control asthma. Includes exercises to aid concentration and relaxation.

Children with Asthma, Second Edition, by Thomas F. Plaut; Pedipress, 1988.
Good advice from practicing physicians with many stories from patients. Easy to read, with glossary of terms and breathing exercises.

The Essential Asthma Book, by François Haas; Charles Scribner & Sons, 1987.
Straight talk about the essential facts every asthmatic should know. Told with no frills, but great clarity. A good overview of the disease.

Hidden Food Allergies, by Steven Astor, M.D.; Avery Publishing Group, 1988.
Provides solid information on discovering and living with food allergies.

Hometown Hero, by Barbara Aiello; Twenty-First Century Books, 1989.
A book of fiction for upper-elementary-grade children, teaching that being different, whether asthmatic or homeless, is a passing condition.

Knight on Horseback, by Ann Rabinowitz; Macmillan Publishing Co., 1987.
A charming story about the "rite of passage," tinged with English history. Knights and kings and an asthmatic young boy rise to meet their challenges.

Luke Has Asthma, Too, by Alison Rogers; Pedipress, 1988.
A gentle story about asthma self-management for the very young reader.

A Parent's Guide to Asthma, by Nancy Sander; Doubleday, 1989.
From the author of "Asthma Newsletter," Nancy relates her daughter's struggle and those of the families she has contacted.

Understanding Asthma: A Blueprint for Breathing, edited by Sheldon Spector, M.D. and Nancy Sander; American College of Allergy and Immunology, 1990.
A collection of articles by various experts in specific fields of asthma: diet, medications, peak flowmetering, among others. This book offers the very latest in suggested practices based on recent research, presented in easy-to-understand language.

INDEX

Breathing
  in evaluating asthma attacks, 26
  exercises, 164–168
  treatments, 159
Bronchial spasm, 8, 17
Bronchodilators, 47–50
Bronkosol breathing treatment, 55

Carbon dioxide, 33
Carpeting, 102
Chambers, 52
Christmas trees, 106
Climate, 24–25
Collections, 102
Common sense, 31–33, 100
Compressors, 56, 97
Conferences, 180
Corticosteroids, 51–53
Coughing, 18, 31, 94–95
Counseling, professional, 41, 147
Cromolyn sodium, 53–54, 153–154

Death, 16, 23–24, 156
Dehydration, 25
Demont, Rick, 44
Doctors
  adding, 39–41
  bills of, 170
  changing, 39–41
  selecting, 36–37
  working with, 38–39
Drugs, 19. See also Medications
Dust, 104–105
Dust mites, 18, 102, 103, 184

Educational resources
  American Lung Association, 178–179
  Asthma & Allergy Foundation of America, 176–178
  conferences, 180
  fun activities, 181
  Mothers of Asthmatics, Inc., 179–180
  National Asthma Education Program, 175–176

Emergency hospitalization, 80–84
Emotions, 1–2, 3–4, 19
Environmental irritants, 18–19, 107
Ephedrine, 44
Epinephrine, 27, 33–34
Evaluation of asthma attacks, 26
Exercise
  benefits of, 154
  breathing, 164–168
  cromolyn sodium and, 153–154
  lung capacity and, 153
  medications and, 153–154
  relaxation, 19, 157–159
  Roosevelt on, 152–153
  Stevens family and, 154–155
  swimming, 154–155

Family
  canceling plans of, 134–135
  chronic illness and, 130
  holiday seasons and, 132–134
  hospitalization and, 66–67
  love and, 141–142
  positive thinking by, 130–132
  quality time with, 140–141
  vacations of, 132
Family history, 14, 22, 63
Finances
  doctor bills, 170
  insurance, 170–172
  medication bills, 170
  Pamela Stevens on, 172
  strain on, 169
  treatment and, 172–173
Fireplaces, 106
Flooring, 102
Food allergies
  of David Stevens, 65
  dealing with, 61–65
  journal keeping of, 88–89
  of Melissa Stevens, 65
  as triggers of asthma, 18
Food and Drug Administration (FDA), 35
Formula substitutes, 32
Fresh-cut flowers and plants, 106
Fresh fruits and vegetables, 106
Friends, 123–127
Fun activities, 181

Furnaces, 106
Furniture, 102

Haas, Dr. François, 153
Hampers, 104
Heart, 30
Hirschsprung's disease, 32
Hives, 63
HMO (Health Maintenance Organization), 171, 172
Hogshead, Nancy, 188
Holbreich, Dr. Mark, 156–157
Holiday seasons, 132–134
Home environment
  airing, 103
  changes in, 105–107
  cleanliness of, 101–104
  comfort control in, 89–92
  common sense approach to, 100
  dust control in, 104–105
  friends and, 127–130
  irritants in, 100
  journal keeping on, 88
  other than own, 92–93
  pets in, 107–108
  reading in, 100–101
  treatment in, 99, 111
Hospitalization
  admission to, 27
  attitude about, 68–69
  charting treatment in, 70
  discharge from, 80
  emergency, 80–84
  family and, 66–67
  feelings about, 67–68
  home touches and, 72–73
  location of bed in, 69
  of Melissa Stevens, 11–12
  Pamela Stevens and, 68, 71, 82
  parents and
    help during, 70–73
    sleeping at, 78–80
  past treatment and, 70
  phone calls during, 73
  presents during, 75–76
  questions during, 76–78
  snacks during, 76
  statistics on, 16
  visitors during, 73–75
House painting, 106
Humor, 10, 149

IgE antibodies, 60
Immunotherapy, 58–61
Industrial pollution, 18–19, 107
Inhalers, 49–50
Insurance, 170–172
Intolerance, 63
Intravenous (IV) medications, 27
Ipecac, 44
Ipratropium bromide, 50, 184–
  185

Journal keeping, 85–89
Joyner-Kersee, Jackie, 188–189

Koch, Bill, 189

Leaves, 107
Lifestyle, 183–184
Linen, 103
Liquids, 25, 94–95
Louganis, Greg, 188
Lungs
  bronchial spasm and, 17
  capacity of, 57, 153
  changes in, 15, 45
  clearing, 160–163
  damage to, 21–22
  in teenage years, 21
  "twitchy" condition of, 94
  weak, 22

Manning, Danny, 189
Marax, 44
Medical data, listing, 116–118
"Medicalese," 39
Medical literature, 14
Medications. See also specific
  names of
  anticholinergic drugs, 50–51
  beta-agonist drugs, 47–50, 153
  bills of, 170
  charting course of, 97–99
  corticosteroids, 51–53
  cromolyn sodium, 53–54, 153–
    154
  of David Stevens, 44
  developments in, 43–44
  effectiveness of, 26–27
  exercise and, 153–154
  future, 184–185

About the Author

MARYANN STEVENS has twenty-five years of experience as the mother of three severely asthmatic children. All three developed asthma in early childhood, continuing into their teens, and all have successfully controlled their asthma. Ms. Stevens worked for eight years in a busy pediatric practice, teaching asthma control classes to adults and children. She is now Supervisory Staff Assistant of the visitors office at the White House. She lives in Virginia.